To the cancer that changed my life for the better…

I'm Still Here!

By

Fatemeh Rezaei Sajadinia

To the cancer that changed my life for the better...
I'm Still Here!

Fatemeh Rezaei Sajadinia

Writing & Design by Sarah Michelle Ritchie

Copyright © 2024 Fatemeh Rezaei Sajadinia

Published by London Book Publishers

All rights reserved.

**To the cancer that changed my life for the better...
I'm Still Here!**

Table of Contents

A Dark Day 1

Beginnings 6

Living with Pain 17

Death, Dying and Surviving 31

Surrounded By Strength 46

Salad and Sixth Sense 61

Oncology and Modern Medicine................................... 71

The Fight: On My Terms 75

To The Cancer That Changed My Life For The Better… 82

    I have learned… 82

    Lesson Number Two.. 83

    Lesson Number Three 83

    Lesson Number Four 84

    Lesson Number Five... 84

Acknowledgements 87

Dr Fatemeh isn't finished yet… 89

**To the cancer that changed my life for the better...
I'm Still Here!**

Disclaimer Notice

The following biography contains information about cancer care and the experiences of one individual affected by cancer.

The experiences shared in this biography are personal and may not reflect everyone's experiences with cancer care.

This information is not intended to serve as medical advice or replace consultation with a qualified healthcare provider.

The author and publisher of this biography are not responsible for any outcomes resulting from the use of the information contained within.

Thank you.

A Dark Day

Where am I?

I am everywhere but here, in this room.

My physical body is here, but not my mind!

I have been sitting here for hours, waiting to be seen, and I don't even know what happened. I was working and felt fine until a few weeks ago. Everything was so normal before I came here—going to work and seeing patients, as I had done for many years. I love it with all my heart, but I can't figure out why I'm sitting here as one of them now.

It all happened so quickly that I didn't even have time to absorb everything.

Nigella, the celebrity chef in all her glossy glory, fills the TV screen in front of us, guiding viewers through different recipes for Christmas. Oh yes, there's not much time left until Christmas, is there? It's funny how things lose and gain significance in times of crisis. Nigella

1

looks so happy and vibrant on the TV, showing the cakes and drinks that fill her festive kitchen. She highlights each step with so much passion. She looks full of life!

Oh God, why is she so happy? Maybe because she's not sitting here on this plastic chair, in this soulless waiting room, terrified of the answers. I envy her right now. I just want to be where she is, doing what she's doing, laughing like she's laughing—I just want someone to take me away from my worries.

I've been worried sick, not knowing what the tests have shown, but I've kept myself busy. Now, time moves so, so slowly—it's unbelievable.

Patients come in and go out continuously, but I am still sitting here, waiting. My appointment was booked for around 9 o'clock this morning, and I was here in good time, so why am I not going in? It's past 11 now, and I am still here, waiting and worrying. I try to find a reason... I was the first one to enter the clinic this morning; in fact, I was there when the secretary opened the clinic's door. I confirmed my appointment with them. Yes, I was definitely one of the first to be seen. So why then, after sitting here for over two hours, am I still waiting?

I'm sure it's not just me overthinking—the nurses have been acting strangely. They keep putting my folder underneath the others; I can see them do it! At times, they look at me and then call someone else in. This is so strange. My heart can't take this anymore; why do I have to go through this? I am a good person. I've always helped others. Why is this happening to me?

The wait is killing me. My hands are sweaty, and I look pale enough to be mistaken for a ghost.

I approach the nurse and ask when it will be my turn to see the specialist. She looks at me and asks if I'm alright. No, I'm not, I say. I've been sitting here for more than two hours. Why is everyone else going in and not me? She says they've been busy and that I'll be seen soon. That's not the answer I'm looking for. "Give me a time, please," I say. "Oh, I'm sorry, but we don't have a specific time; you'll be in soon," she replies.

Oh God, she doesn't understand me! No one seems to understand me these days. I've been waiting desperately for this appointment. I haven't had a proper night's sleep since 13th October, and today is the 22nd. And here I am, still waiting for the test result. It's driving me mad.

Looking around the room, no one else seems to be as upset as I am. Women are sitting calmly, reading books or playing with their phones while waiting to be called in. How is it that it's just me waiting for the big news?

I scan the room for a sad face, hoping to feel less alone in my suffering. But unbelievably, I don't find any. This is the first time in my life I've ever wanted to see someone suffering. I've always wished happiness for others, but now I feel so desperately lonely. That's who I am—I help people feel better—and so I recognise what I'm doing now. I'm looking for comfort, for a connection in a shared experience.

Despite what I see, I know the truth. I keep repeating to myself: *You're not the only one. Look around. Look at these women—they've had their treatment and returned to normal life. You're not alone.*

I'm in the strangest state of mind. There's really no experience like this. Sitting here, thinking about my life, it feels as though I'm in a cinema, watching a film about myself. I'm the main character, but I haven't seen the whole script yet.

Why have I reached this point? Where did I go wrong?

This isn't the first time I've fallen ill, but this feels different. Still, I remind myself: I've never let any illness bring me to my knees before. I can deal with this one, too.

And then my name is called…

To the cancer that changed my life for the better…
I'm Still Here!

Beginnings

I was born in 1964, under the Iranian sun, to parents who had longed for a girl. Before me came ten boys, five of whom tragically lost their short lives during or shortly after delivery. During her pregnancy with me—her 11th—my mother was told I was measuring so large that she was put on a special diet to reduce my size and lessen the likelihood of complications during labour. A large baby is often a sign of a healthy baby, so my parents must have been expecting smooth sailing. Unfortunately, life had other plans.

Because I had been so longed for, my family celebrated my impending arrival in our home in Tehran with a grand party that lasted seven days and seven nights. There was plentiful food, thanks to my affluent businessman father, and guests brought gifts of money, declaring me a blessing. But when I was born, it became clear I was not a healthy baby. I was failing to thrive, unable to gain weight, and constantly unwell. On top of being weak, I was plagued by what were likely viral infections and other ailments. I sometimes wonder now if my mother's diet during pregnancy left me malnourished or caused some lasting damage. Whatever the cause, it marked the beginning of a long battle with my health.

When I was two years and two months old, my parents had my sister, bringing our household to a cosy nine members. I have a vivid memory from around that time of my mother being heavily pregnant during one of our regular holidays to the north of Iran. We often visited close friends while we were there. On one such visit, I recall my mother being in excruciating pain. The grown-ups acted swiftly, rushing her to the car and leaving me with a feeling of confusion and fear I can still remember vividly.

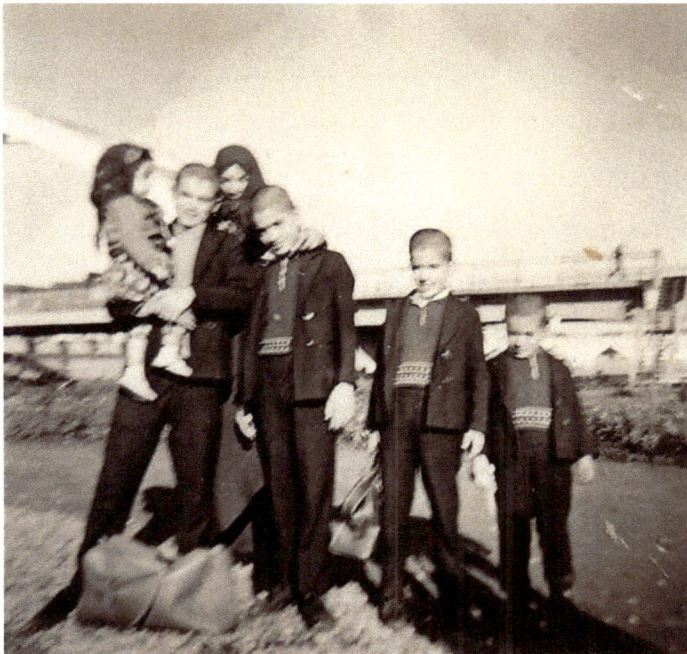

My mother, brothers and me; (from left to right) Javad holding me,

with Hossein next to him followed by Hasan and Amir,

posing on holiday in North Iran.

7

To the cancer that changed my life for the better...
I'm Still Here!

In my memory, my mother is seated in the middle of the back seat, with me on her right side, wide-eyed and innocent, watching as she moaned in pain and wrung her hands incessantly. Her friend sat on her left, reassuring her and comforting her as best she could during the drive to the hospital. This memory is so vivid to me, I can still feel the fear even now. At the time, I obviously didn't understand what was happening, but the emotions were very real. I often think about the messages this experience conveyed to me and the parallels with situations I would encounter later in life.

As I grew, I had my head in everything. I was the curious child who wanted to know how things worked and wouldn't rest until I had at least tried to figure it out. I remember investigating the washing machine to see how it worked and breaking things apart around the house to satisfy my insatiable curiosity. Luckily, I was so loved and accepted that I didn't get into too much trouble.

All of my brothers doted on me. Hossein, in particular, went out of his way to make me happy and show his love for me. He would comb my hair and pick flowers to adorn it. I felt cherished—a pretty princess! Then my sister came along and declared herself the queen, wanting to be the centre of everything. When we played, I'd have my turn and then be sent off to help around the house, but her turns always seemed endless!

She was headstrong—she knew what she wanted, and she made sure to get it.

Our beautiful old house, where I was born, had a large pond in the middle and two grand staircases—one leading to the kitchen and the other to a landing—that connected the yard to the building. When I was around five or six years old, we moved to a new house. This traditional Iranian-style home had a driveway, an outdoor toilet, and a lovely front yard with a pond and a miniature flower bed. My father, who had a natural affinity for gardening, adored the flower garden. He would plant fresh basil, cucumbers, tomatoes, and wildflowers in abundance.

Inside, the house had a spacious lobby to greet visitors. To the left of the lobby were two living rooms, and at the end of the house was a simple kitchen with a small patio. Upstairs, a landing led to a toilet and bathroom, and further up were two rooms. Finally, there was one last staircase leading to the fifth and final room. It was just enough space for all nine of us!

I loved our new house. Without distractions like TV or mobile phones, we spent time together, talking, playing, and simply being with one another. I remember having such a large family that there was always someone around to keep me company.

When we eventually got our first TV, I was around eight years old, and it caused quite a stir! This was before the Iranian Revolution, so everything on TV was uncensored. My father worried about us being exposed to anything inappropriate, so at first, he forbade us from watching it altogether.

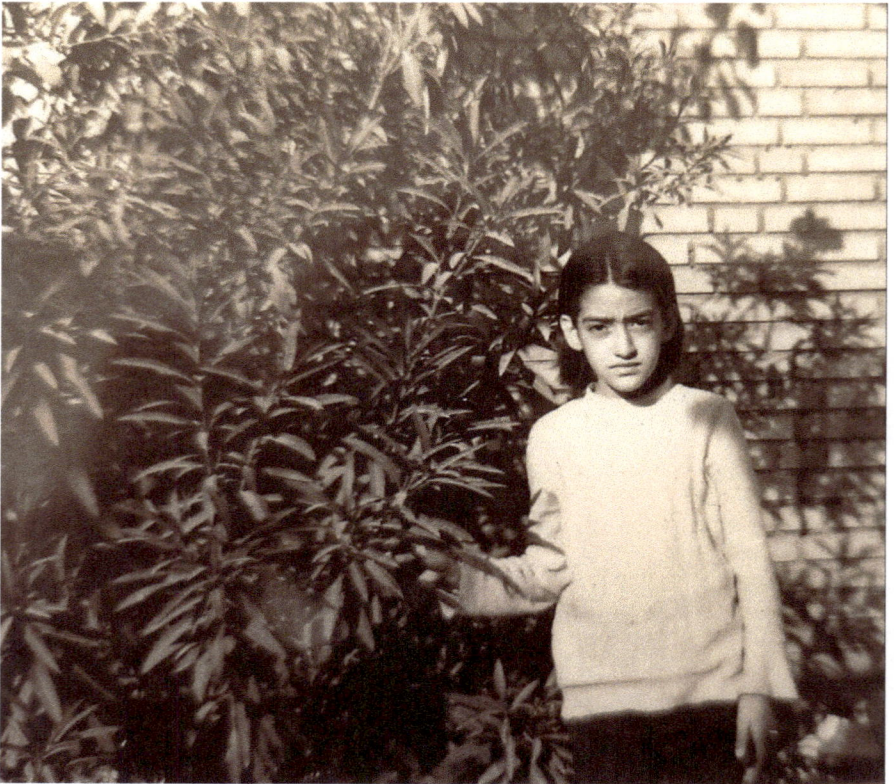

Me, aged seven or eight;
an ordinary girl with so many questions for God.

My brothers, despite having decided they didn't want us girls to watch anything (such were the prevailing cultural attitudes of the time), would find ways to get around the TV ban, and we'd be roped into helping! The TV was housed on the top floor, in that final room. When my father was out, my five brothers would sit in that room, huddled together to watch the impossibly small screen set into its chunky plastic casing. I would be stationed on the first-floor landing, poised for action at a moment's notice, while my sister would be similarly waiting on the ground-floor landing. Each time my father returned, we'd run our respective relay legs to warn my brothers to get out and avoid trouble. Looking back, it must have been a funny sight, but they always got away with it—thanks to us girls.

In our family, it was expected that daughters were polite and helpful to their mother, while boys were eager to learn and helpful to their father, and so it was. My father had sold one of his businesses to buy the new house and now drove a truck for a living, so it was important that everybody pulled their weight. I started to help out more around the house, leaving very little time to play. I would sweep two and a half floors, wash my brothers' socks, repair clothing, help my mother cook meals, and generally have a hand in everything. This earned me the nickname '*Everybody*,' because I was always doing something for someone.

I was still curious and desperate to understand how everything worked, so I took up sewing—making curtains and bedroom sets—and baking all sorts of things in our very basic kitchen. When I did play, I'd take my one dolly and play healer; it was all I ever wanted to do. It was the same at school—I was driven to help others, even while achieving good results in my own work.

Meanwhile, my fourth-born brother, Hassan, was very, very ill. He was suffering from a kidney problem and had to go to the hospital regularly. I remember my mum crying every day, worrying herself sick about him, so I stepped up again and made sure everybody else was looked after. Each day, I'd cook and make sure everyone was ready for school, work, and university, despite my own ongoing weakness and susceptibility to illness.

At the time, my eldest brother, Reza, was a medical student and took charge of looking after me. I'd been prescribed antibiotic (penicillin) injections, which I had once a week from the age of eight, eventually moving to once a month for a whole year. My family had been told that, without these injections, any simple illness could kill me. My immune system was so low that it could lead to rheumatoid arthritis in the future.

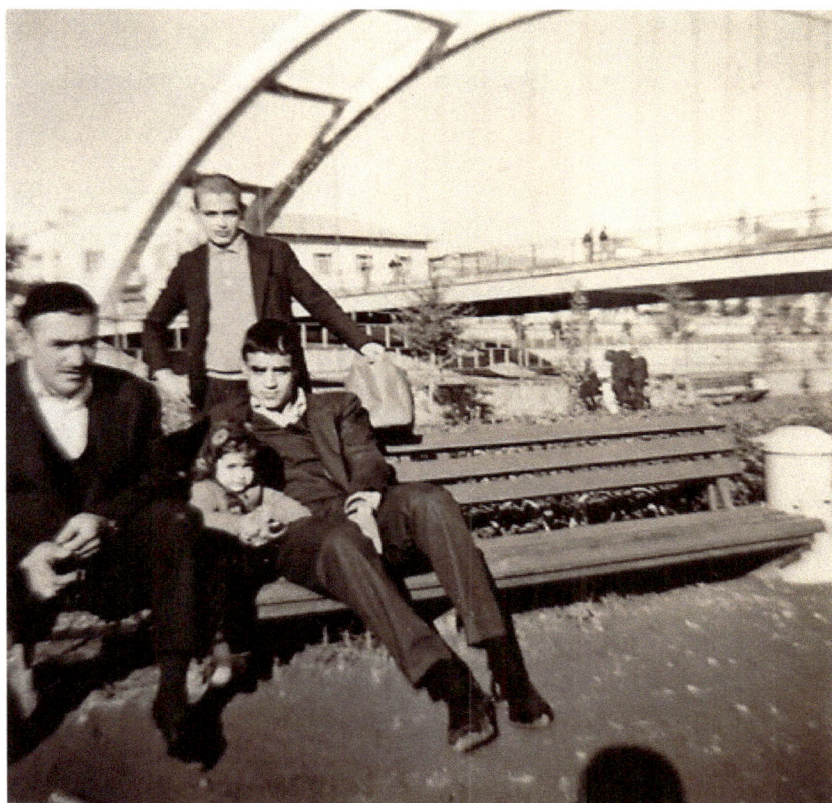

My father, me and my brothers: Reza and Javad.

I remember being utterly terrified of those injections, but my brother was resolute in his dedication. He'd sit in one of the first-floor rooms, carefully preparing everything. A small metal bath would be placed over a fire to boil the syringe, the sight and smell of it was enough to send me into hiding. My brothers, Hasan and Amir, were tasked with finding me and dragging me out from my various hiding spots.

To the cancer that changed my life for the better…
I'm Still Here!

I became an expert at disappearing. Sometimes I'd wedge myself into the cupboards, other times I'd sneak out onto the patio behind the kitchen. One of my favourite spots was the empty pond, which we used as a storage space. I'd crouch there, trembling, as my brothers searched for me. Being so small and skinny, I could squeeze into almost any corner. But no matter how clever I thought I was, they always found me.

Every time, they'd try to reassure me. "It'll only be a few seconds," they'd promise. "You're so strong; you can do this. We're so proud of you." Their words were full of love, but they couldn't ease my terror. I'd resist with every ounce of my strength as they pulled me towards that room. Hossein, who couldn't bear to see me upset, would slip away before the ordeal began, his love for me making it too painful to witness.

In the room, I'd be confronted by the sight of the syringe boiling in the bath. I'd shake with fear, knowing what was coming. Eventually, though, I'd give in. They'd lay me out on the daybed—a makeshift couch made of mattresses, duvets, and blankets—and hold me in place. One brother would hold my hands, the other my feet. Reza, the master negotiator, would make me promises to soothe me. "I'll get you some delicious chicken afterwards," he'd bargain. "Your dudush is looking after you, don't worry." He'd even promise a ride in his fancy Peykan Javanan car to Andre's, the best salami maker in Iran at the time. Their

14

sandwiches and fried chicken were my favourites, but even the thought of them couldn't completely outweigh the dread of the needle.

Looking back, the love I feel for my family is overwhelming. It must have been so hard for them to go through this with me, seeing my distress. Yet they never wavered. Not once. They all came together to care for me, to make sure I got through it. I was so loved, so lucky to be surrounded by such staunch devotion.

Our house also had a rooftop that we accessed from the topmost room—the one where the TV was. In the summer, we'd often sleep up there, all of us snuggled together under the open sky. As a child, I would lie on my back, gazing up at the stars. My mother would encourage me to ask God my questions. To this day, I still look to the stars when I seek wisdom or guidance. Back then, I'd ask why I became so ill, so often. I'd ask why I had to suffer, why I couldn't just enjoy my life like the others did. I'd wonder why I had to miss out on parties and the usual fun that children experience. My life always seemed filled with pain, and all I wanted was to be normal. I'd plead for answers under the stars, every time, but I was always met with silence.

I know now that if I had been given an answer, it would have been that all of this was to make me strong, to prepare me for a life as a healer. After all, how could I possibly help others to the fullest if I didn't understand what they were going through and how it felt?

To that little girl, pleading for answers, life seemed very unfair.

Living with Pain

For some, the country air is as normal as the city smog is to others. For me, it was pain and sickness that were normal, woven into my daily routines and clinging to all my experiences. In my earlier days, they were my constant companions in one form or another, and my teenage years were no exception.

When I began my periods, they were instantly painful, and each month they only grew worse. It was almost impossible to do ordinary things and simply get on with life when the pain plagued me so relentlessly. Once again, my life was shaped by pain, and the things I could do were limited. However, thanks to my parents' and brother's support and love, I had survived my tumultuous early years and learned how to cope. There were no counsellors to help me, nor were there others like me who could empathise. It was just me, trying my best to be a good and helpful child, striving to make the most of things. So, I continued to work hard, throwing myself into every opportunity that came my way, and life went on, even during those horrendous times of the month.

At school, I was excelling. Like a sponge, I absorbed knowledge from every person and every corner of every room. I was particularly good at the sciences and maths—so much so that my friends and classmates would clamour for my attention and guidance. I would teach them everything I had learned after we'd sat in the same class because, according to them, I always explained it better than the teachers. I sometimes wonder if they had any idea what life was like for me outside the classroom, and if they did, would it have changed anything?

Despite my weakness, I was good at sports. I ran faster than my classmates and excelled at volleyball. Back then, we had house sports teams and an official school team that competed against neighbouring schools nationally, and if we were good enough, internationally. I was honoured and so proud to have been picked for the school team. Unfortunately for me, my father was old-fashioned and wouldn't hear of me exposing my legs to the world by wearing the shorts required for the team. I was disappointed, but I had faced enough disappointment already; I knew how to cope.

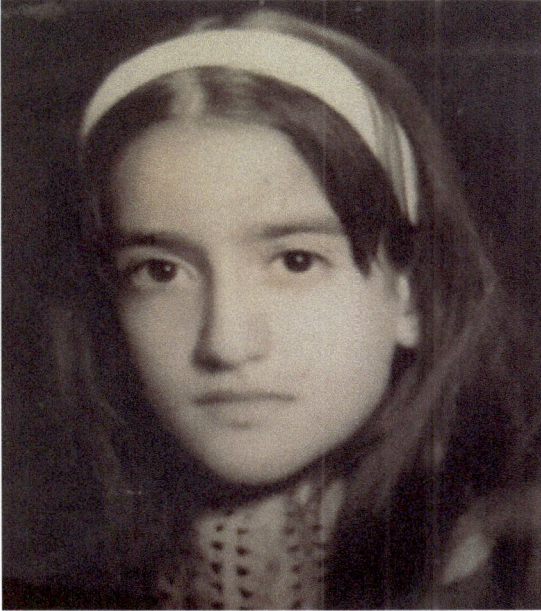

Me around the age of ten or eleven,
having been selected for the school volleyball team.

Surprisingly, Reza had seemingly fallen out of love with medicine and moved to the UK to study Economic Analysis shortly after I turned 12. There, he met his wife, and my other brother, Hossein, joined him shortly after. My mother, of course, mourned the loss of her sons to another country. Her sadness at our scattered family was palpable; she missed them so much. Then, the Iranian Revolution began the year I turned 15, and not long after it ended, Reza returned to Iran with his wife and young child.

To the cancer that changed my life for the better…
I'm Still Here!

I was just finishing Year 10 in high school, completing the equivalent of British GCSEs, when they moved back and settled on the second floor of our family home. The house now felt wonderfully full of life, with Amir in the little room on the third floor and me on the ground floor with my younger sister, in a room divided into two by a giant wardrobe separating us from my parents.

School continued to be a wonderful gift for me. It was a place where I could satisfy my curiosity and share the gift of knowledge with others. After my A-levels, I wanted to continue my education and go to university to maintain the momentum and feed my hungry mind. My mother supported me wholeheartedly and had countless conversations with my father, trying to convince him of the value of a university education. She spoke about how bright I was and the opportunities that could open up for me. For me, learning felt as vital as oxygen—I simply wouldn't be satisfied without it.

However, my father was set in his ways and had, at times, even been displeased with me attending school. He wanted me to become a calligrapher, and as the head of the household, his decision was final. So, with little choice in the matter, I studied calligraphy for around two and a half years. Yet, it wasn't enough for me. To satisfy my curiosity, I also took up hairstyling and beauty as hobbies.

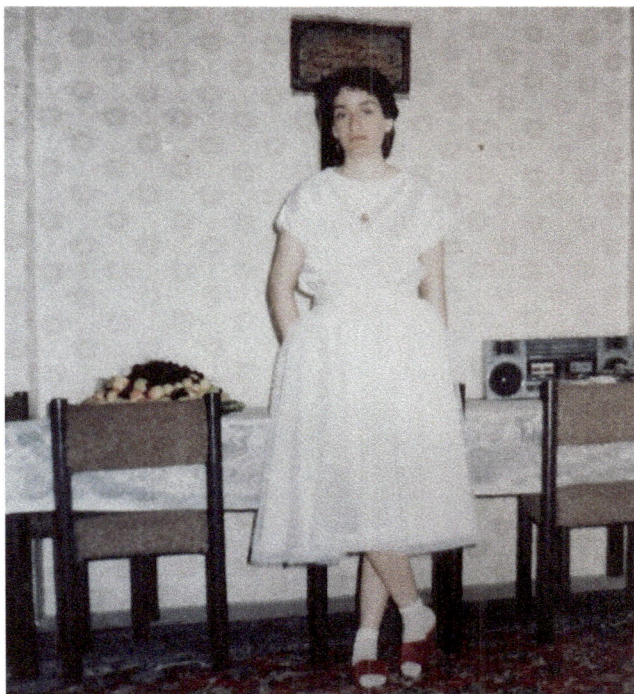

Me, aged 18, proudly wearing a dress I'd made myself.

Then, when I turned 19, Reza became my saviour once again. During a conversation, he told me, "You're good, you're talented—go and find yourself." He helped by introducing me to friends of his who worked in national TV. Before long, I was working as a researcher for film and TV characters from 8 a.m. to 1 p.m. every day. At the same time, Reza's lovely wife, an editor at the newspaper *The Tehran Times*, gave me a job as her research assistant, thanks to my excellent touch-typing skills. For the next five years, I worked at the TV network in the mornings and then walked two hours to the newspaper, starting at 3 p.m.

and finishing around 10 p.m., after which I'd take a taxi home to my waiting father, who would inevitably ask, "Is this a suitable time for a young girl to come in?"

I flourished during this golden period of my life. I was happy, with high job satisfaction and Reza's unyielding support and level-headed guidance. While my other brothers had been content to follow my father's traditional beliefs, which often meant restricting my activities and even stopping me from going out, Reza understood my desire to explore the world and live a fulfilled life.

I still lived side by side with pain, but I didn't let it stop me. My work received constant praise, I saved money, and eventually, I bought myself a car. I was proud to support myself and follow through on my choices. I became the family's big achiever—none of my female cousins in my generation had accomplished what I had, and I shone brightly, like a diamond.

During this time, I took up sports again, joining the Iranian women's running team—and I was good! I worked out regularly, determined to be as fit and healthy as possible, even though back pain began to feature more and more in my life. Then, at the age of 23, my life changed one day when the doorbell rang while I was home alone.

Little did I know that on the other side of the door stood a man who would change my life, enriching it with unconditional love and support. I went to answer the door.

Quickly fetching my head covering, as culture dictated, I opened the door to a tall man wearing a smart brown suit and tie. I glanced briefly at his handsome face before asking, "How can I help you?" He asked if Amir was at home, to which I replied, "No, but can I take a message?" The handsome stranger smiled and said, "Just tell him your cousin was here, and I was hoping to go for our tickets today." I knew Amir was planning to pick up visa applications from Turkey, but I hadn't known who he'd be going with.

To the cancer that changed my life for the better…
I'm Still Here!

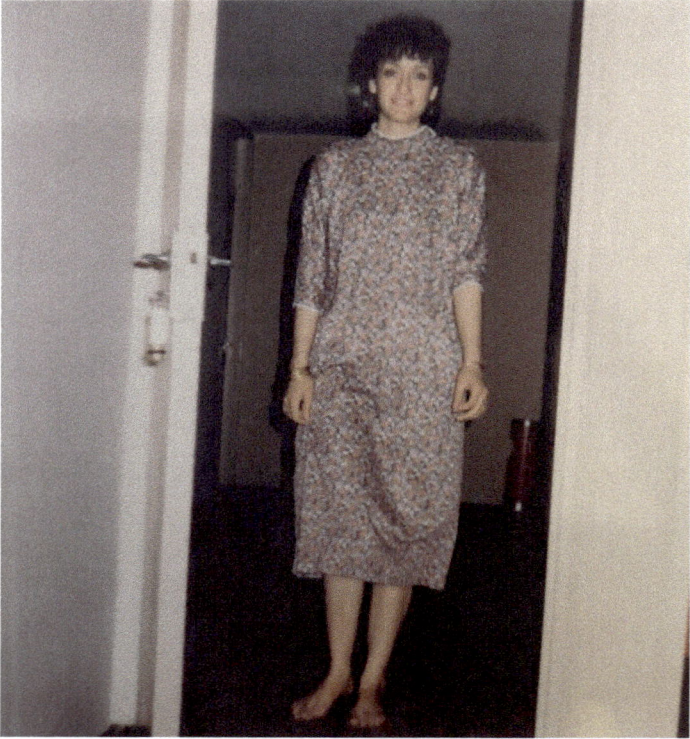

Me, aged 23, tall and slim, wearing another of my handmade creations.

I was shocked. I'd never met this man before. "Cousin? You're… my cousin?" I had a huge family, with countless first, second, and even third cousins, but I was certain I'd never met Mohammad—except perhaps when we were very young. Our busy lives had kept us from knowing each other, from seeing each other grow or celebrating our respective achievements. And now, here he stood, making my heart flutter, utterly disarming me with love at first sight—a love that would last a lifetime.

When our courtship became common knowledge, everyone was stunned. I'd always been so preoccupied with my health, so determined and driven in my career, and so absorbed by life's distractions that I'd never even looked at boys, let alone thought about love.

It began with us exchanging written messages, delivered by his youngest brother, who was only 14 or 15 at the time. This went on for a few months before we officially became a couple.

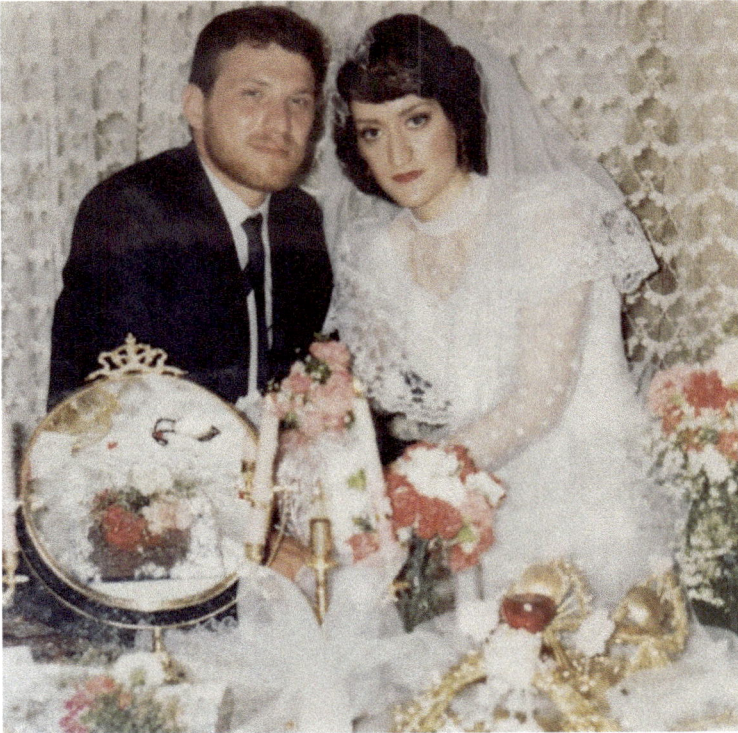

We married for a love that still grows stronger each day.

To the cancer that changed my life for the better...
I'm Still Here!

Mohammad and I wed in Iran in April 1987, embarking on married life with hope for our shared future. Despite the back pain that plagued me early in our marriage, we quickly learned to listen to one another, made efforts to understand each other, and grew to compromise. It became our privilege to make each other happy.

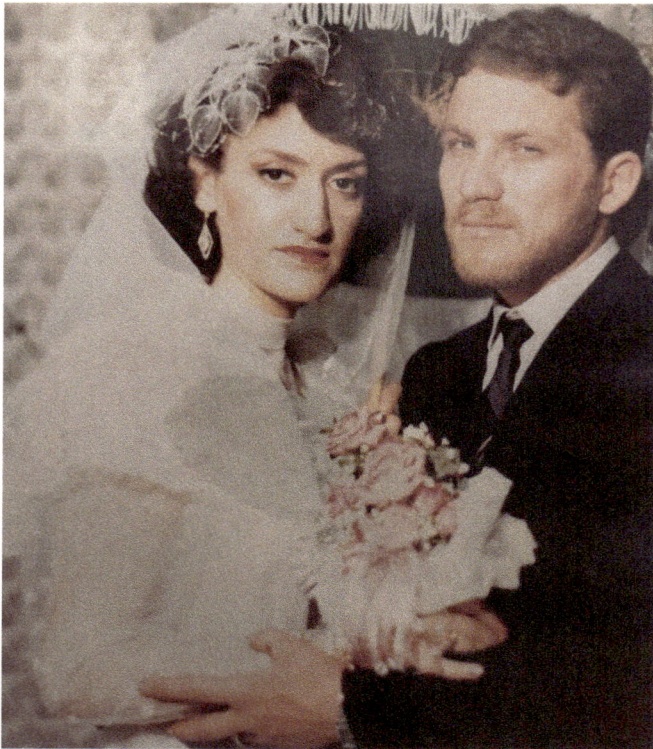

Me and Mohammad on our wedding day - we couldn't have guessed how much we'd be going through together.

We made it work, despite Mohammad being traditional and me a free spirit, shaped by my father's strict upbringing. I had already proven I could make sound choices for myself, and I wouldn't be satisfied with restrictions placed upon me. This led to some clashes early in our marriage but also gave us the chance to learn from one another. Together, we grew into better versions of ourselves.

I had my daughter in 1989 while visiting the UK, and I instantly fell in love again—and then once more, after the birth of my son two years later. Motherhood allowed me to love, care for, and help another person in ways that soothed my soul. But, even with this wonderful life, my pain persisted.

Shortly after my son's birth, my back pain became severe. My ever-patient husband tirelessly drove me to countless doctors, trying treatment after treatment. Yet, after giving birth a second time, the pain grew unbearable. When my son was just under a year old, I was admitted to hospital for an operation on my back.

To the cancer that changed my life for the better...
I'm Still Here!

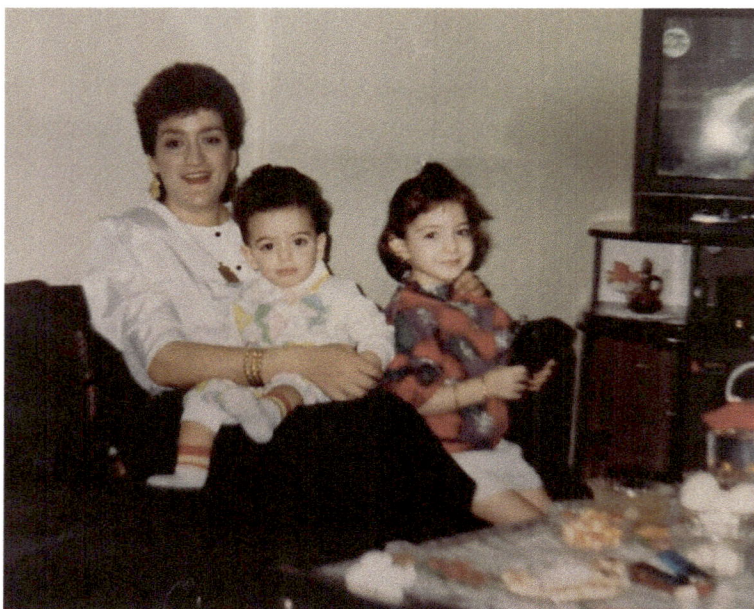

Me and my children. My daughter Hanieh,
aged nearly three and my son Hamid, a few months old.

The hospital was private, with one of the best surgeons in Iran at the time willing to operate on me to ease my pain. It cost a small fortune. However, in those days, medical professionals in Iran rarely communicated with patients as they do today. I didn't fully understand what procedure awaited me in the operating theatre. Still, I had my faith to comfort me and an unwavering hope that I might emerge on the other side with less pain, so I went ahead.

The operation was successful in the surgeon's terms—he performed a spinal fusion, fixing two vertebrae together with metal screws. I was told this would severely restrict my movement, preventing certain bends and ruling out my beloved running. Suddenly, I was hearing, "You can't do that," and it had all been done without my full understanding or consent. I wasn't sure I would have agreed had I known the lasting effects on my life.

Unsurprisingly, I was devastated. I questioned my choices and wept. To the little girl who had once pleaded for answers from the stars, this was yet another blow—another way life had been upended. But, as always, I resolved to dig deep and overcome the challenge.

I quickly decided to pick myself up, turning my focus to helping others. My devastation transformed into curiosity, and I became determined to understand what had happened to me and what I could do about it. Once I had recovered enough from the operation, I began studying exercise and sports therapy. Within nine months, I achieved my fitness instructor qualifications at levels 1, 2, and 3.

Armed with this new knowledge, I took my first step towards healing others, teaching exercises to help ease their pain. Yet, my own

To the cancer that changed my life for the better...
I'm Still Here!

pain lingered, driving me forward. I couldn't rest—I needed to learn more.

Fatemeh Rezaei Sajadinia

Death, Dying and Surviving

In 1998, I was granted a conditional visa to live in the UK following a visit to my already-settled brothers. Almost immediately, I applied for a Higher Education Foundation Course (HEFC) and passed IELTS—a rigorous course designed for English as a second language learners, covering reading, writing, speaking, listening, and more, enabling access to higher education. I excelled in my HEFC modules, achieving 100% in every test, and was even interviewed and featured in *Oxford Magazine*. All of this, while settling my family into a new culture with a new language and traditions, made for a tough and busy time.

When I completed my courses, I found myself at a crossroads. My love of learning and my life of pain had always coexisted, but since my fusion, the quiet, nagging urge to understand myself had only grown louder. Still, I wasn't sure what path to take. I sought advice from a friend, an Iranian GP, and asked him what he thought I should dedicate my university studies, career, and future to. His answer made perfect sense: he suggested physiotherapy. He explained it would help me understand my own anatomy and come to terms with what had happened to my back. Something inside me lit up—I knew he was right, and I started applying.

To the cancer that changed my life for the better…
I'm Still Here!

To my delight, I was accepted by three universities, including Northumbria, which offered me a full bursary. This life-changing offer filled me and my supporters with joy. In 1999, I embarked on the next step of my journey, determined to achieve my goals. I worked tirelessly and relied on my own determination, even though my brothers, well-established in their careers, were close by and eager to help. As always, I sought independence and the pride that came with achieving things on my own.

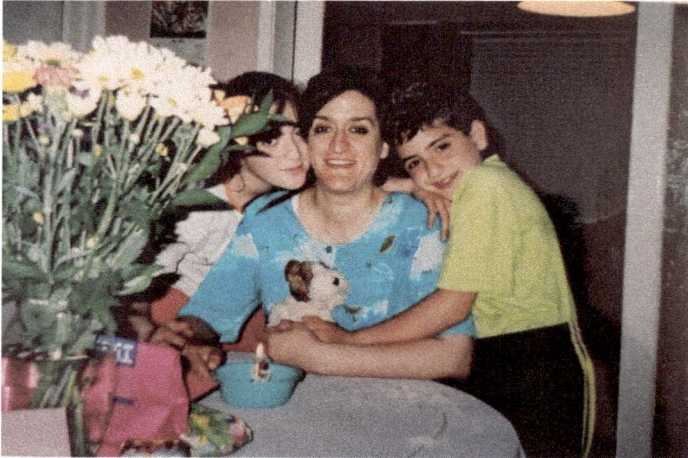

Me, Hanieh and Hamid, in our first year in the UK:
They had no idea how hard mum and dad were working to look after them.

When I wasn't at uni three days a week, I walked four miles from Gateshead to Newcastle to cut hair for the Iranian community, charging £2 a cut. Thanks to the extra training I'd done back in Iran, I was in high demand. I also worked as an interpreter, supporting Farsi-speaking children in English schools. The pay was low, but every penny helped during those days. When I wasn't studying, interpreting, or cutting hair, I was caring for my family, doing my best to teach my children everything they'd need to settle happily into UK life. My days were utterly packed! To complicate matters, Mohammad worked late evenings at a pizza shop, so for three years we crossed paths like ships in the night.

The first year of uni flew by in a blur of enthusiasm and activity. Each assignment boosted my confidence, though it was never easy. Without the internet at home, I had to make constant trips to the library, copying everything by hand—books and paper were everywhere at home! Just before my second year, my lovely brother Hossein gifted me a little Honda Accord to show his support and encourage me to keep going. I felt proud to drive to uni, and life began to shift a little.

However, when the second year began, life's challenges started piling up. Both Mohammad's and my mothers were unwell, far away in Iran. My children were still struggling with the language barrier, and the stress of it all weighed heavily on us. On top of this, Mohammad and I couldn't support each other as we'd have liked due to our commitments. Unsurprisingly, I became overwhelmed.

One day, it all came to a head. Despite my bursary, high rent and mounting financial worries left me feeling cornered. I decided the only solution was to give up my beloved degree. Painstakingly, I wrote a letter to my tutor, explaining I couldn't cope and had to abandon my dreams.

I hand-delivered the letter, and as it was being read, I sat and cried. My tutor, John, was surprised. He reminded me I was doing well, but I explained I was barely holding on. I told him I had no choice but to work and couldn't manage both. Calmly, John reassured me, saying the university was there for me. He suggested I take a couple of weeks off to rest and think things over. True to his word, he called me regularly to check on how I was doing.

His kindness and belief in me were priceless, giving me the strength to carry on. I returned to uni and persisted.

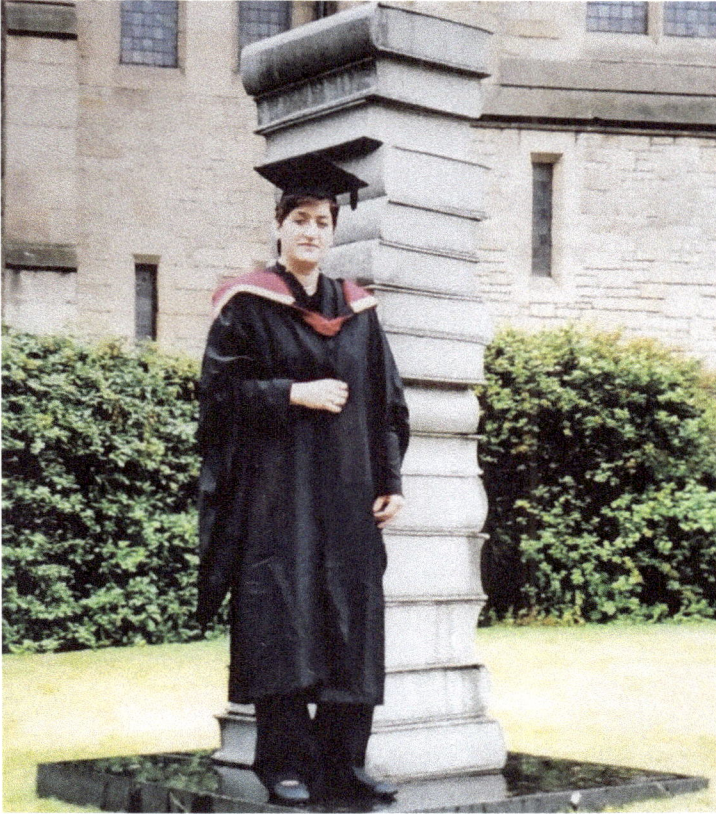

Graduation day, summer 2002, aged 38. I completed my BSc in physio, with pride.

I achieved my degree through sheer hard work and unwavering passion. In the process, I realised I had accomplished more than I initially set out to do. Not only did I gain a deeper understanding of my own condition, but I also reignited my desire to be a healer.

Soon after, I began working at the Queen Elizabeth Hospital Trust in Gateshead, where I was honoured to help people move and feel better every day. I stayed with the trust for three years, gaining invaluable experience and creating wonderful memories before taking the leap into the private sector—the next chapter of my journey.

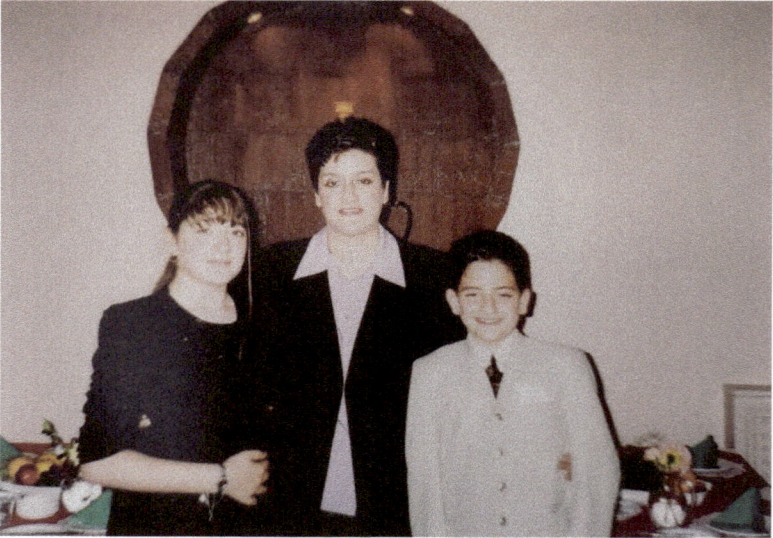

My children and me, partying at Amir's restaurant, celebrating my graduation.

All the while, the painful periods I had long suffered still persisted in the background of my days. Then, in 2006, they reached a crescendo and almost crippled me. I was living and working at a clinic in Newcastle at that time, and money was still an issue for us. I wanted to start my own business but convinced myself to wait for the right moment when things were perfect. Then, I was diagnosed with endometriosis, and in October or November of that year, my doctor told me I needed a total hysterectomy or I could be in serious trouble. I didn't overthink it; the thought of getting rid of the pain was enough, so I agreed.

Shortly after sunrise on the 11th of January, 2007, I was taken down to the operating theatre to have a full hysterectomy. It was supposed to be routine. It was supposed to take only two and a half hours…

My family had taken me to the hospital, settled me in, and waited with me. They then stayed in the waiting area while I had this simple procedure carried out. I fully expected to wake up in a few hours, with everything having gone as planned. *Life isn't always what we expect, though, is it?!*

When I woke up, it was dark, and I knew instantly that something wasn't right. I had been under anaesthesia for longer than a couple of hours, it seemed, and the amount of tubing and wires everywhere shocked me. I looked around at my family, and the horror hit me full force. My children were crying, and Mohammad looked lost and vulnerable: this was serious.

I soon learned I had died on the operating table, having lost far too much blood. Usually, surgeons expect blood loss of up to 200 millilitres during a full hysterectomy, but what they found when they looked inside me was that the adhesion between my gut and womb – the stickiness that had been restricting and painful all these years – was far more severe than they had first thought. As a consequence, they had to remove a section of my gut, and because of this, I lost more than 2 litres of blood that day, more than half the total blood volume in my body. I was told there was a 20-second period where I was clinically dead, but the team worked hard to transfuse me, and luckily, they brought me back. I was then transferred to the ICU after my operation, and that's where I woke up after losing a whole day. I stayed in hospital for five more days and had another two blood transfusions during that time because doctors were still concerned about my haemoglobin levels.

Then, one night, while I was still in recovery on the ward, I was uncharacteristically restless. Sleep evaded me no matter what I tried, and despite the sedatives I'd been prescribed, my mind refused to switch off. All of a sudden, I felt a shift in the air, and a sort of image appeared in front of me. It wasn't a clear image like you'd see in person, or in a photo, but one that's almost indescribable with words. It might have been light, a person, a feeling, or a combination of all three. I suppose it was more of an awareness, on my part, of a presence which I felt strongly was bringing a message for me. Whatever was happening in that moment was trying to communicate: I was being reminded I'd been given a second chance at life.

In the days after my operation, I began to bleed, similarly to my monthly periods, which should've been impossible, and this went on for 70 days straight. I didn't understand all of this, and neither did many of the professionals I saw, so I was back and forth to the hospital, where I was admitted on a few occasions and even taken back into the operating theatre for further investigations. This was a frightening time. Nobody seemed to understand what was happening, least of all me. I was drained and losing so much weight throughout it all. That second chance seemed so far away now; I really felt as if I was dying.

The bleeding eventually stopped, but the bad news didn't stop coming. Not long after I'd gone home for the first time after my operation, I received a heartbreaking phone call from a relative in Iran. My auntie had sadly passed away, and we would need to break the news to my mother, who had been almost inseparable from her for as long as I could remember.

Almost immediately, a sense of guilt rose inside me, and questions started to gnaw away at me: *she hadn't been ill, so why did she die and not me? Had she taken my place? Was this because of me?*

To the cancer that changed my life for the better…
I'm Still Here!

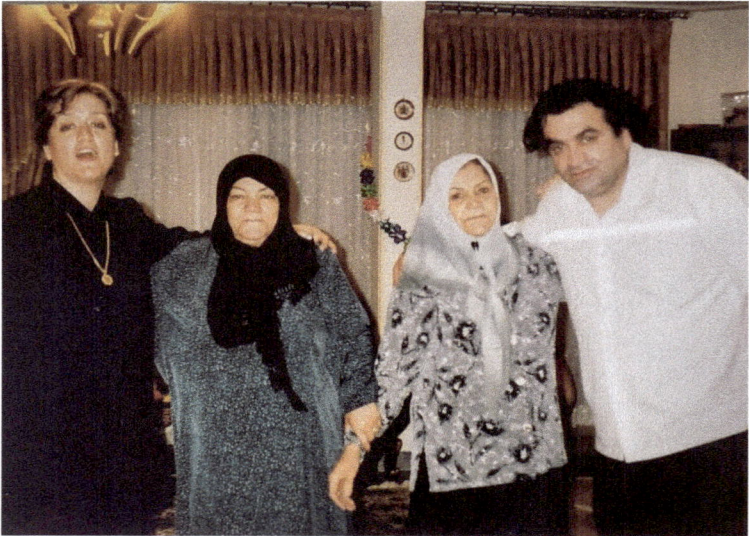

Me, Mum, my auntie and my youngest brother,
Amir at my surprise 40th party in Iran. Mum holds on to her dearest sister.

The Iranian New Year is on the 21st of March. On the 23rd, despite everything I had recently been through, I invited everyone over for a celebration. This was something I enjoyed doing every year: cooking up a feast for my loved ones, though I had to have a little help this year. Happily, my mother had come over from Iran to join in our celebrations, but it wasn't long before I noticed something was wrong. I could hear her talking from across the room, and to me, there was something about her voice that sounded off. I was overcome by a deep sense of foreboding.

My mother's voice was unusually raspy, so I approached her and asked why her voice had changed. She told me she didn't know and that she was fine, but I wasn't placated. I looked at her, standing in front of me. For as long as I could remember, my mother had worn a scarf around her neck, and today, it was a beautiful white scarf. I asked if I could lift the scarf and look at her neck, and she tried further to convince me that there was nothing to worry about. Eventually, she told me there was a little something there (under her scarf) that had been there for a few months and that she'd had it checked out in Iran. I lifted the scarf and saw a visible lump.

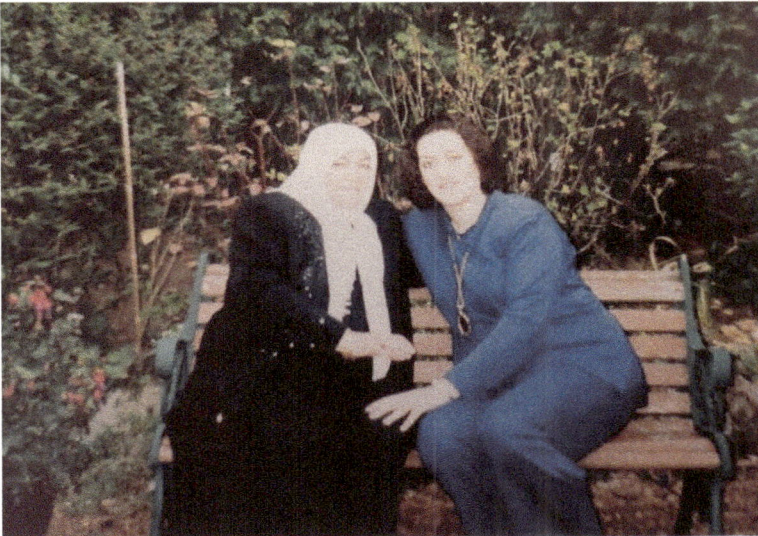

Me and mum, with her beautiful white scarf around her neck.
She loved nature and was her happiest in nature.

To the cancer that changed my life for the better...
I'm Still Here!

I told my mother she needed to go to a hospital, and so she did that day, on the 23rd of March. Then, on the 27th of March, she was diagnosed with an aggressive cancer. I tried to remain positive, thinking through all the options we could take, but an inner voice was rushing me. It was a sort of sixth sense, the same voice that had guided me toward uncovering the knowledge I needed to understand my body and its illnesses. Only this time, the voice was louder and clearer than it had ever been: I had the strongest sense of running out of time.

The hospital told us that my mother would likely live for another two years. So, with this in mind, Hossein planned to take her to Iran by private jet, so she could be at home, comfortable in her own surroundings. I felt strongly that she wouldn't make it back home; my inner voice was even more sure of it, claiming she would pass within two weeks. Sadly, I was right. My mother died on a Sunday evening, on the 22nd of April, around three weeks after her diagnosis, in the UK.

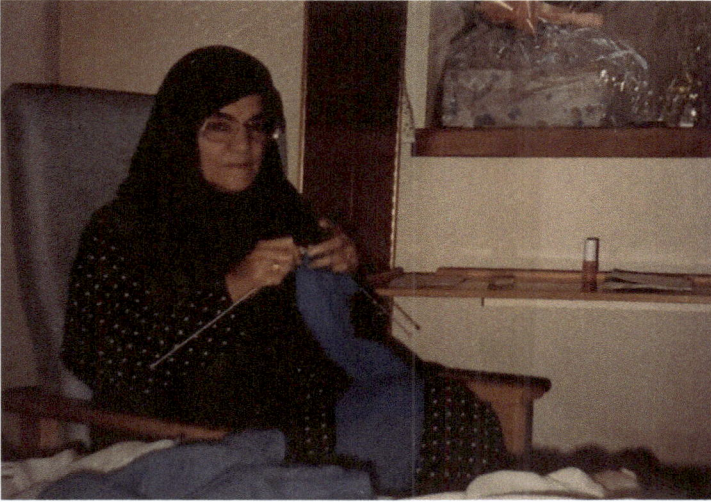

Bless her, mum was always in hospital. This time she was in Gateshead, UK.

Understandably, this hit me so hard. I fell into the same pattern of thinking as I had after my aunt's death: I really felt that she had taken my place, that she had died because I had lived, and these thoughts took me to a really dark place. I couldn't understand why, when I had been the one plagued all these years, I hadn't been the one to die.

We took my mother home to Iran to be buried. Reza, Hossein, Amir, and I sat in the aeroplane and travelled with her. She was buried on my 20th wedding anniversary, surrounded by her family and their boundless love. I was struggling emotionally. My own physical trauma, followed by the loss of my auntie and mother in such quick succession, left me reeling. I couldn't believe it was possible for a human to go through so much, so quickly, and come out the other side. Even though there was so much to do in the early days following my mother's death (all the usual sorting and tending to things), and even though I had my brothers and Mohammad to help and support me, I was still spiralling emotionally. Grieving was a waking nightmare.

Back in the UK, I felt such a profound loss. Life would never be the same, but I knew somehow that I needed to go on. I decided to try to fill the space and refocused on my doctorate that I had begun completing online. I didn't stop to try to deal with my grief, trauma, and stress. I was a healer, and there was still healing to be done.

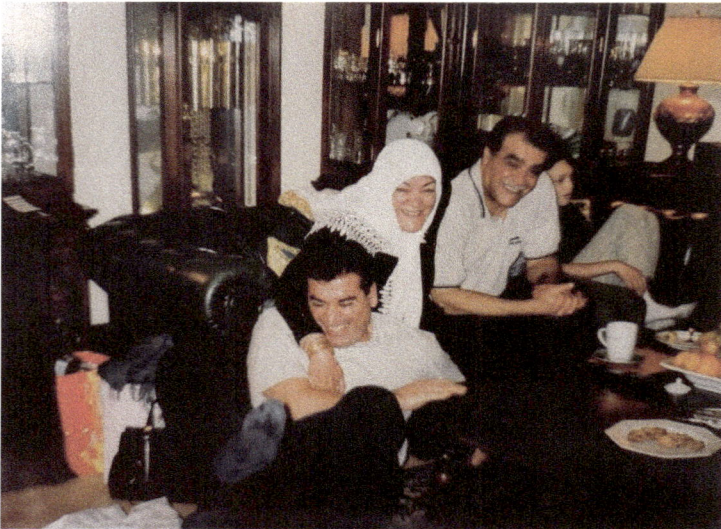

Mum's happiest times were when surrounded by her children.
Here, she's tickling Hossein, while sitting next to Reza.

Of course, life did go on, and then, in 2010, I was awarded my hard-earned doctorate. Armed with confidence, I decided this was it! It felt like I had reached the pinnacle of my life. I had survived, and more than that, I had thrived and moved forward in my life and career. I needed to grab this momentum with both hands, so I decided we needed to move to London for a fresh start – and we did.

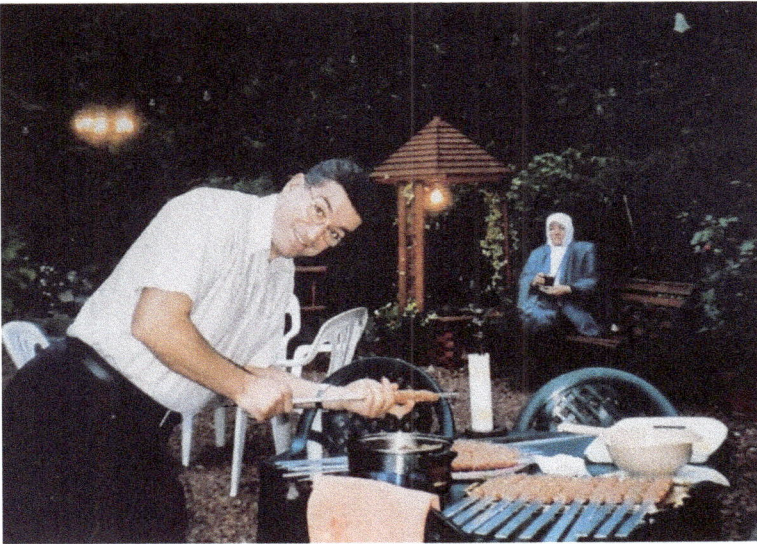

The most kind-hearted person I know, my Hossein, cooking and looking after everyone, with mum happily enjoying the scenery.

To the cancer that changed my life for the better...
I'm Still Here!

Surrounded By Strength

The majority of women in the Western world, following a hysterectomy or during menopause, have access to, or are prescribed, HRT. I was no exception, and I took it as prescribed for eight years, without so much as a single check-up to see how my body was reacting. During these years, I had so much to contend with, to overcome, and to achieve that I didn't stop to check in with myself and see how things were going. Unfortunately, inside me, the worst was happening, and I had no idea.

Life in London was good. Mohammad and I were still incredibly in love. We had date nights where we'd go to my beloved Oxford Street and enjoy each other's company over a burger. We were also so proud of my children, who were growing into such beautiful people. I was truly content.

I noticed something wrong in my right breast in the summer of 2015. There was a change in the hardness when I compared it to my left breast, so in September, I was sent for a mammogram. Just three weeks later, on the 13th of October, I was sent for an ultrasound scan. I had arrived on my own, after finishing my shift at the hospital, because I hadn't taken it that seriously yet, unlike my work. I thought, *this'll be fine; I'm worrying about nothing.*

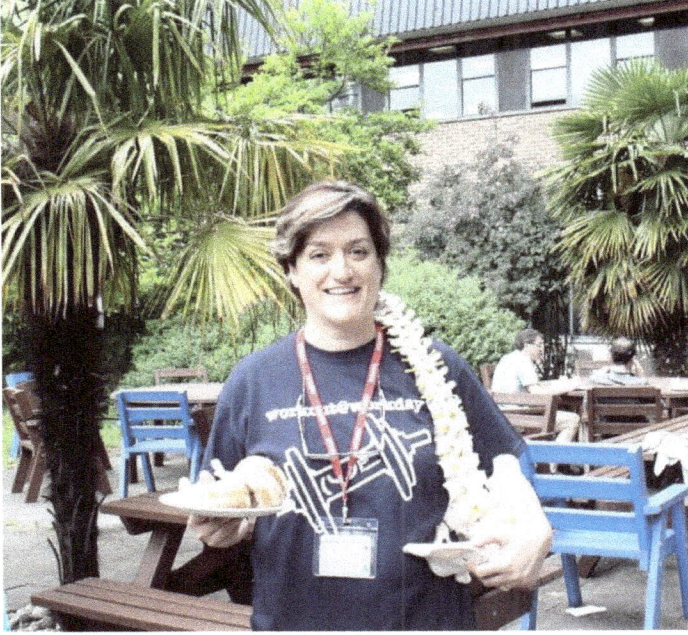

Here I am, dedicated to my healing work.

So, there I was, in my white physiotherapy uniform, thinking that I'd be in and out and on my way in no time. But, as before, life had other plans. As I lay on the bed, the technician looked at my scan, and her expression gave me the first hint that things were not okay. Shortly after, another staff member joined us, and I saw them glance at each other — only briefly, but it was definitely there. Did they think I couldn't see them?

It was over soon enough, and I couldn't wait to be alone with my thoughts. Then, as I tried to leave that appointment, I was stopped in the corridor and told I needed to have an urgent biopsy before I left. There was no choice. As I lay back down on the bed, I gritted my teeth through the pain. There was no one to hold my hand as the needle went in, and no comforting words as three samples were taken for the lab. I was alone — just me and my silent tears. This wasn't going to be straightforward.

Afterwards, I was given lots of information about cancer, without anything actually being said. There were lots of maybes and possibilities, but certainly no solid confirmation of anything. This left me bewildered: *did I have cancer? Was there still hope that I didn't?* I now know I was being prepared.

I sat alone in the car following the appointment, for what seemed like an eternity, all the while wondering why I saw shock and worry on the faces of the doctors and nurses, who must do this all the time. I could feel their sense of urgency, but there were no words of comfort for me, no full explanations of what was happening, no transparency. I almost felt like I was being treated as a child — one too delicate to know the horrid truth, too inexperienced to make good choices — and it almost made me panic. Of course, I pulled myself together, started the engine, and drove. Somehow, I made it through the next couple of weeks.

One day, the phone rang with an appointment for me. Then came that dark day on the 22nd of October, 2015, when I sat in a hospital waiting room for three incredibly long, lonely hours, thinking, *'This won't happen to me, it can't! I'm a good person, it doesn't happen to people like me...'*

Mohammad was by my side the whole time, but I'm sure for him it was a similarly lonely, terrifying set of moments, played out as if we were watching actors on a film set. We saw women arrive after us, and we saw them go through for their appointments. This only added to my sense of desperation: I'd waited for this appointment, prepared myself, and now I felt like it was being dangled in front of me — the proverbial carrot, just out of reach.

Eventually, I was called into a small room, where we were greeted by a doctor, a tall man with worry lines etched deeply into the well-worn skin behind his glasses. I thought about how those lines signalled all the bad news he'd had to deliver over the years, and I wondered if they were about to get deeper. I asked for my results straight away, but he insisted we have a current ultrasound before we discussed anything.

**To the cancer that changed my life for the better...
I'm Still Here!**

During the ultrasound, I saw the man's face fill with another layer of concern, and I knew something was majorly wrong. He asked if I'd been told about this, to which I replied no, and he was shocked.

Eventually, he turned to me and said, *"It's not good news. You've got a cancerous tumour in your right breast, and it's about six centimetres in diameter."* Of course, I had seen the evidence, but I'd been in denial, assuring myself it was just fatty tissue. He continued, *"The bad news is, it's spread under your right arm, and there are already a few lymph nodes involved, so it's not a good situation."*

My breath caught in my throat, and I looked down, struggling to digest all of this. A wave of a hundred emotions crashed over me. *"If it's so bad, why have you been keeping me waiting out there for so long?"* I pleaded. My doctor answered me honestly, *"This is so bad, we were readying ourselves to tell you."*

I thought back to Nigella on the TV, all glossy hair, beaming her way through her festive recipes, without a care in the world. I thought about the doctors huddled in the corridor, finding the task ahead of them so tough. Then I thought about myself, sat waiting to find out my fate. *How did they think this was for me? How did they think my day was going?*

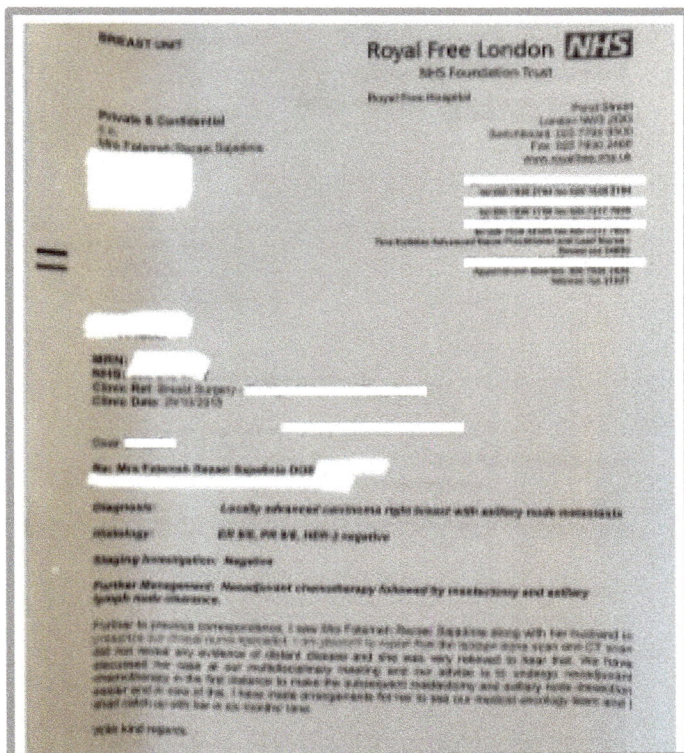

My letter from the breast clinic

I remember asking my doctor what would happen next, and I was told I'd be sent for further tests to check if the cancer had spread anywhere else. I was then given a blue card with the word 'URGENT' emblazoned across the top. On the card was a list of all the things I would face in the coming weeks, including a nuclear medicine test, MRI, and other tests that would see my entire body investigated for signs of cancer.

I asked what would happen after that, and he told me that if it hadn't spread anywhere else, it could be treatable with a double mastectomy, clearing both underarms, courses of chemotherapy, and a potential course of radiotherapy. He said all that would likely take two to three years. Immediately, I asked how long I might survive afterward, and the answer chilled me to the bone: "Maybe five years or a little more."

There was a thunderous roaring in my ears, my lungs screamed out for air, and the room spun uncontrollably. Instantly, the sums didn't add up for me. Ahead of me, I saw years of intense trauma that would ravage my body and numb my soul in the name of treatment, and all I'd get out of it was a few more years. A few more years with what was left of me, after putting myself through that. I caught sight of my beloved husband on my left side. Through my own tears, I could see his fear as he tried to absorb this news.

My URGENT blue appointment card

I took a deep breath and asked, "What if I don't want to do that?" My doctor replied, "You don't have any other option." So, that was that. My future was mapped out, reflecting my past pain and suffering, all the way to an early death. I didn't know it then, but my doctor was fighting his own battle with cancer behind the scenes, while spending day after day with other sufferers. Sadly, he went on to die a year after our first meeting.

At the end of my appointment, my doctor referred me to the oncology department at the Royal Free Hospital and told me I'd hopefully be seen there the following week. I was then ushered towards a small room opposite the one we were in, where I was introduced to the Macmillan nurses. As I knew, this was end-of-life care: it was now confirmed—life as I knew it was over for me. I had literally just received a death sentence.

One nurse held my hand when I sat down, as you might hold the hand of an upset child. They were talking, but my ears had stopped hearing. I looked around, bewildered, but my eyes weren't seeing properly through the tears. All I could think about was my poor, poor children and husband.

Somehow, I left that room, managed to leave the hospital, and ended up in my car. I couldn't stop thinking about the absurdity of it all. Just yesterday, I'd been working and, even now, I still felt fine. Why had they been talking as if I were actively dying? But I couldn't even finish these thoughts before my phone started ringing with appointments. I was shocked at the speed of it all. It was coming faster than I'd ever thought possible, and it was all so final. I tried to breathe and realised I needed space to deal with this news, and time to come to terms with what I had learned.

We drove home with my tears accompanying us the whole way. When we arrived, I went straight to my bedroom and shut myself away for hours. I needed to think about how to support my children, how to break the news to my beloved family, and what would happen to my patients who relied on me. I was consumed with thoughts of how this would affect everyone else, being the healer that I was. I felt so desperately alone, despite the concern on my children's faces and that look in my husband's eyes.

I thought about Mohammad, who was bereft. It was so hard seeing his hopes and dreams dashed in the space of an appointment. Though he said all the right things to me, and I knew he'd be there as much as he could, I felt the urge to lift him back up. But I was weaker now, I needed support. When we spoke later, he told me he'd reached out to my brother, Hossein, because he knew we had a special relationship and his messages would be powerful for me. Ironically, Hossein's very good friend had recently gone through a similar scenario and was currently undergoing similar treatment: I had been there for him, so we knew he would understand.

To the cancer that changed my life for the better…
I'm Still Here!

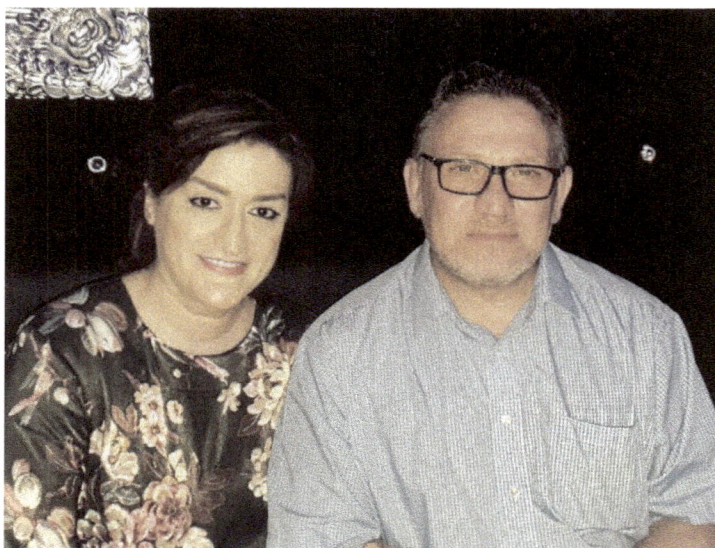

Me and my Mohammad.

That evening, Mohammad took me out in the hopes he could raise my spirits a little. Unfortunately, it was an evening I won't ever forget. Back in the good days, we'd go out to Oxford Street, feel the buzz of the shoppers and revellers mixing all around us and enjoy each other's company. On that evening, it was almost as if we were in a parallel universe. I felt extreme loneliness among the crowds of normal people here. Everything felt out of place, almost unreal. My gaze was downcast and the tears, though silent, flowed freely. Mohammad would stop to ask about buying things in the shops we loved, but all I wanted to know was who would care for my children; *what would happen to them?*

Mohammad repeatedly told me, "It'll all be ok", simple words, spoken from his hopeful heart, and I realised then that he was reassuring me in a way I hadn't experienced since my diagnosis. This was a sentiment so completely different from what I had confirmed by the medical professionals, that it felt odd, hearing words of hope. I couldn't know how important his words were then, but it was absolutely what I needed to hear; someone believed in me, someone saw a way I could survive this, someone helped me to hang on… bless my husband!

Following that night out, with a thousand conflicting thoughts and feelings jostling for space in my traumatised mind, I asked my husband for some space; I just needed to get my head together. Of course, he let me be alone for a while, but I couldn't stop thinking about what I might've done wrong: *What wrong choices might I have made? Why had this happened to me?* I spent a lot of time remembering my past and the whole of my life leading up to that dark day.

Undoubtedly, from the 22nd to the 29th October, 2015 was the most horrific week of my life. I couldn't face work, but I couldn't tell them why either. I felt this was a very private time, while I struggled to come to terms with things. Unfortunately, it was easy for Mohammad's supportive words to get lost in all the many negatives. I was left without hope, given all I'd been told. Not once had alternatives been offered to me. Not once was I encouraged to fight, even during that week when I had so many phone calls back and forth and attended so many appointments, that all my tests were quickly completed and it was confirmed to have not spread anywhere else.

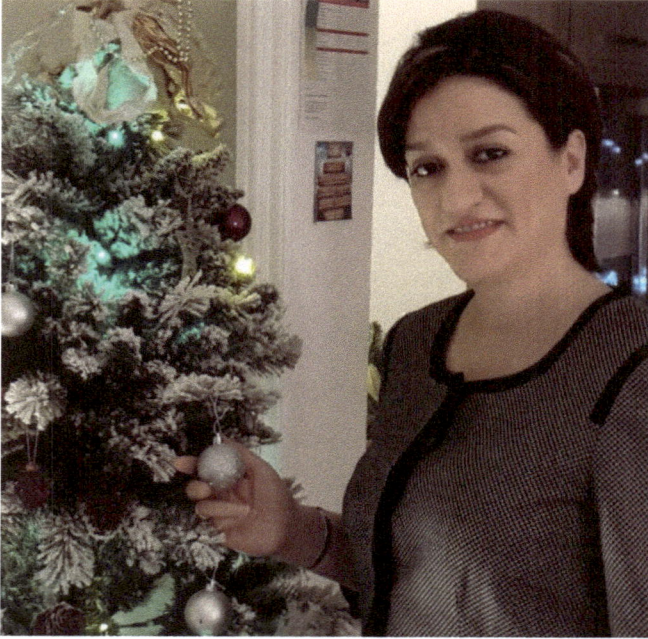

Keeping a happy mask on, while getting ready for a TV show in London,
after being invited as a guest expert on back pain

Then Hossein called me and asked me a question I hadn't yet been asked, a question seemingly so simple, yet so heavily loaded: "What do you want to do?" I didn't know it at the time, but just hearing those words leave his lips, hearing them puncture the air between us, would kickstart a change within me. He, like my husband, hadn't confirmed the death sentence I'd been handed at the hospital but had opened my mind to other possibilities and, importantly, to hope.

I told Hossein that I didn't know what to do. He asked me what the hospital had said, and all at once the terrifying words came tumbling out. I told him how scared I was and how I didn't want to put my children through what had been decided for me, especially when the short-term effects would so heavily outweigh any long-term gains. Hossein listened to my every word patiently, and after a while, he said the words that changed my life forever: "You don't have to, Fatemeh, there are other ways."

Something clicked when he spoke that sentence. A light switched on, and the curious inner child woke up inside me. She began to wonder…

What else could I do?

Hossein went on to promise that he would help me in every way he could. He'd already collected a wealth of information in support of his friend's own diagnosis, and now he would be there for me, in every way possible.

Hossein told me, "My beautiful sister, this is not the end of the world. So many people have survived cancer."

I came away from that phone call with a new perspective. Finally, the positivity of my husband and brother started to outweigh the negativity I'd so far experienced, and I felt a flicker of hope.

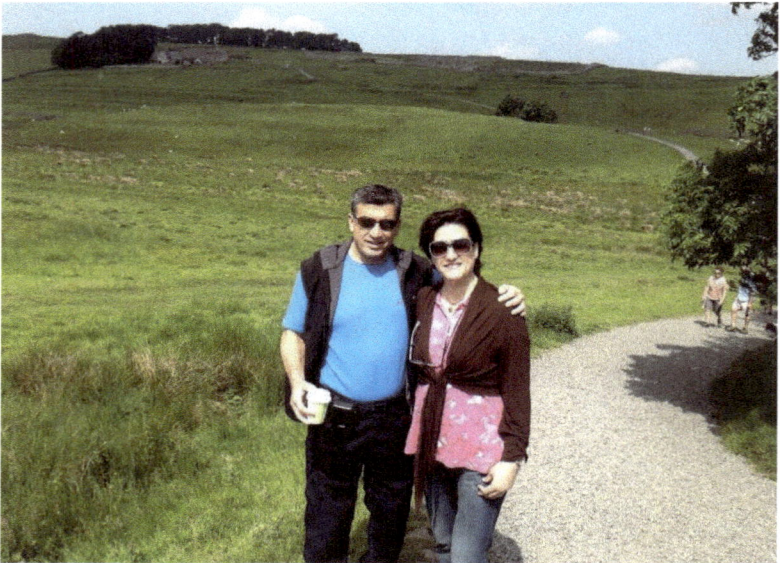

Hossein and me at Hadrian's Wall,
pumping my energy up after my diagnosis in the North East.

Salad and Sixth Sense

After my phone call with Hossein, I felt excited. Now I had the belief of those closest to me supporting my decisions, and the knowledge that there were other options available to me, besides the medical processes offered. In the space of that phone call, I'd had a complete shift in perspective; I didn't feel helpless anymore!

I went online and looked at the website Hossein recommended, *The Truth About Cancer*. Immediately, I was thrilled to see so much varied and well-researched information all in one place. There were videos, recipes, articles, and books about so many cancer-related topics, including tons of complementary and alternative therapies. There was also a whole community of people empowering themselves and each other in their own fight against cancer, and I immediately felt the absence of judgement. I also found an acceptance of people following their own path toward healing, whether that be through modern medicine, by using alternatives alongside modern medicine, or even therapies in the absence of it.

I began to think about food again and soon found myself almost on autopilot, preparing a salad. This was not me; I was not a salad type of person. But I made my vibrant, colourful salad by sheer instinct, and from that moment, with the trust in myself to follow that instinct, I began to fight.

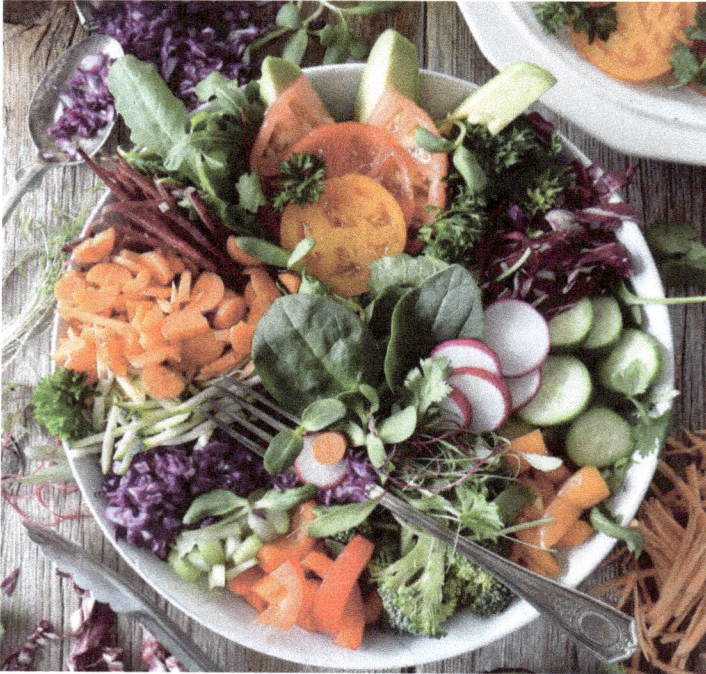

Wholesome, nutritious foods are what I craved.

I began eating my salads on Friday and continued through Saturday and Sunday, eating nothing else. I didn't know why I was so driven towards this food, but I had the feeling that following my gut was the right thing to do. Mohammad marvelled at the change in me, and on the following Friday, he suggested another trip to Oxford Street. This time, I felt the old familiar excitement, so off we went.

One of the hallmarks of our usual visits to Oxford Street was enjoying a good burger together. I usually had a pretty average Western diet, and burgers were among my favourites. But when I thought about having a burger that night, for some unknown reason, it just didn't appeal to me anymore. We went back on Saturday and Sunday too, and I still instinctively avoided the burgers. Other than food, the world was back to how it had always been – full of life and possibilities.

Believe it or not, by Sunday evening, I felt full of energy and somehow like I was breathing better. I hadn't had any symptoms affecting my breathing, so to speak, but all of a sudden, I could just breathe better! What I didn't know at the time was that an extremely important switch had been flipped by Hossein in one quick moment, and now my mind and body were working in connection to learn new patterns of behaviour to take me forward safely and successfully. I couldn't know just how important this would be.

On the very next Monday, the 26th of October, we had to go back to the hospital for another scan. I didn't want to go, so I tried to delay things by going to a coffee shop first. We found one easily, sat near the hospital, and had a bite to eat. Here, surprisingly to me, I felt like I wanted to eat bread, so I chose a toasted chicken and avocado sandwich, with a coffee to help it down. Surprisingly, that sandwich made me feel so good; the texture of the bread – so soft, the taste – so sweet. I had to ask what it was: 'Just an ordinary wholemeal slice!' But after days of the same salad, my senses were sparking, and I felt so alive just sitting there, chewing and smiling.

Afterwards, at the clinic, my fearful tears returned once again, but as I took a seat, hope coursed through my veins and a thousand silent prayers for all of this to be over escaped with every shallow breath I took. I'd been trying so hard, and I hoped for good news.

On this second visit, the wait was much shorter than on that dark day. Straight away, I was told there was good news, and for a brief moment, I hoped with every inch of my soul that my cancer had disappeared, or maybe my results had been mistaken in the first place? But the good news was the confirmation that my cancer hadn't spread, other than to the three lymph nodes I already knew about, and my inflammatory markers were slightly down.

The same doctor as before reiterated what my treatment plan had to entail, but a little hope remained, so I spoke up and told him I'd been eating salad. Sternly, he told me, "No, you can't treat a six-centimetre tumour by eating salad." He confirmed that, while what I was doing was fine, it had to be done alongside my treatment plan.

There was an orange on his desk, which he picked up, presented to me, and told me, "It's this big. Treat this cancer while it's treatable." I asked him what he meant. After all, I'd received a death sentence the last time I saw him. Shockingly, he said, "There is a small chance that you might survive for longer, after all the treatments."

Through my veil of tears, I asked what else I could do for myself, to which he replied, "There's really nothing you can do. The only way you will have a life is if you follow the treatment plan."

I felt let down, confused, and deeply unsettled by the words and treatments I'd received so far, rather than the hopeful, excited buzz I'd been experiencing while trying my own things. By that time, it had only been nine days since my diagnosis, and I hadn't even told everyone about it yet, though my children now knew.

So, when I came home from that appointment, obviously saddened and once again afraid, my son told me about his friend's mum, who was a gynaecological surgeon. He had made an appointment for me to go speak with her, so my husband took me to her beautiful, big home the next afternoon. This doctor was beautifully dressed and clearly successful, I noticed, as she sat opposite me in the kitchen. The equally beautiful cat sat eyeing us from his position on the breakfast bar.

She spoke first. "I'm sorry about your diagnosis. My son told me, and I am sorry, but unfortunately, it is what it is." I wonder if the shock was visible on my face. This woman was so upfront and matter-of-fact. I gathered myself and meekly asked her, "Isn't there anything else I could do about it?" To which she replied, matter-of-factly, "No, even with all the treatment you've been offered, you may only have about two to five years to live." I very nearly fell to the floor as her words hit like shards of glass; I was defeated in that moment. Couldn't she have given me some hope? Why had she agreed to see me, just to tell me these same things?

The tears returned, and the hope I'd felt before I'd gone to that appointment, and before I came here, was less of a beam now, more of a faint flicker, and it was threatening to go out. In the car outside this lady's house, I sat in the dark, next to my husband, silently remarking once again on the death sentence hanging over my head. I had to really try not to give up.

Then a remarkable thing happened. Nazanin rang me. She was a physiotherapy graduate from Germany, who had found me on the internet in 2011/2012 and asked me to do an adaptation period with her in London. I helped her successfully register with the HCPC, and she had been so grateful, always expressing her desire to repay me in some way.

Nazy called me while I sat in the car, tears streaming down my face, and I had to ask her to call back. She wanted to know what was wrong; she could tell I was crying and wouldn't respond favourably to my attempts to push her away. I told her everything and heard her own voice catch in her throat as she listened to my frustration over my lack of choices and fading hope. Then Nazy told me she was sure there were other ways.

Nazy had achieved a degree in chemistry in Iran before switching her studies to physiotherapy in Germany, so she had knowledge that I didn't. Like Mohammad and Hossein, she too supported me in wanting to try other things, reinforcing my budding belief that I didn't have to be a helpless victim, and I began to feel powerful again. The first thing she brought me were bitter almonds, which contain natural cancer-fighting elements. Next, she brought me frankincense essential oils to massage into my skin, which also contained cancer-fighting properties, and I started to use both regularly.

Over the next few days, my instincts drove more of my decisions. I reinforced the things Nazy was telling me by using the *Truth About Cancer* website, and I quickly grew in knowledge and confidence. At one point, feeling empowered and having built up a good amount of trust in my instincts, I tasted the frankincense oil. I was driven to ingest it, and so I did! Within me, bricks of hope began to form an armoury tower, and I was climbing to the top of it; the fight was on!

Although I returned to work, Nazanin continued to visit me two or three times a month throughout it all. She would give me massages, bring me remedies, and keep me company. I was truly blessed to have had her come into my life. Hossein also continued to support me. He had always been there for me, unequivocally. In fact, I almost found it a little strange how he just seemed to know the right things to say and do whenever I needed him, but he did. To me, he had always been a giant of a man—someone I not only looked up to but felt protected by—and I counted myself very lucky to have him there with me on the front line.

One day, Hossein introduced me to a juicing book that revolutionised my thoughts and feelings around food. I was drawn to this book, and I soon learned about the nutrients and properties of foods, such as the fact that a green juice, including spinach and other cruciferous vegetables, can detox and boost energy levels. So, after I had read up on all the benefits of juicing, I decided to go all in, and Mohammad dutifully went out while I was at work and shopped for everything I needed to get started.

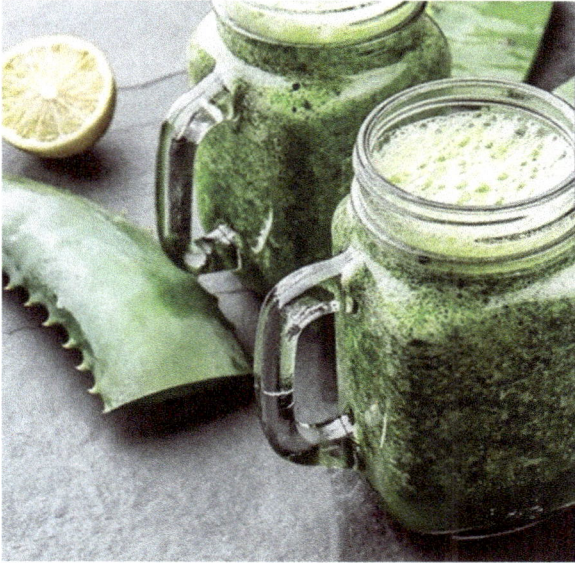

My recipes and my husband's juicing, kept me going strong.

I had begun to treat my body, so for the first seven days, I drank five different juices per day, each a different colour of the rainbow. I consumed no other food at all. After that first week, I had a short break where I ate normally, before doing another week of juicing. I went on like this for six months: one week of juicing, then one of normal eating. During that time, I had never felt so good—I felt energetic and optimistic!

I continued using frankincense oil, and I studied meditation, herbal medicines, and medicinal foods for good measure. I was committed to doing better for myself! I didn't know it then, but because my beliefs had been challenged and changed, a whole new world was opening up to me.

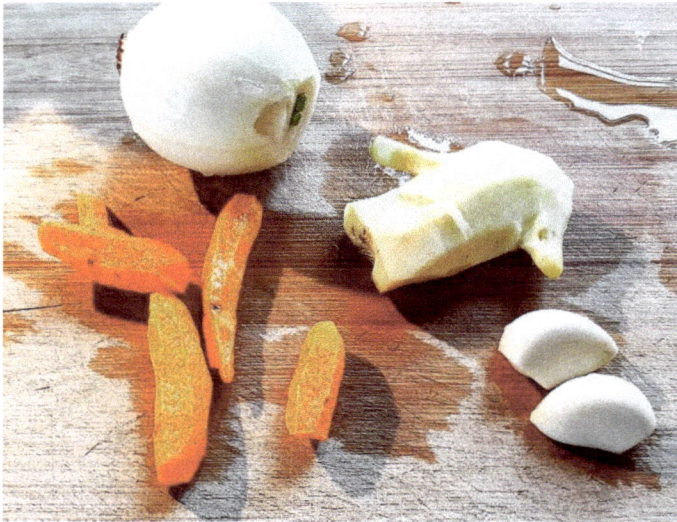

I kept fresh ingredients within my reach at all times

Oncology and Modern Medicine

Thank goodness for the kindness of the people in my life, the ones who were helping me, for I needed them more than ever after my oncology appointment.

At that time, I was still juicing, enjoying the benefits it brought me and believing in the goodness it was doing for my physical health. My hopes grew with each passing day. But as the time approached, I knew I didn't want to attend the appointment. I felt that I had come so far, feeling so good on my own, and then everything went dark again when I thought about speaking to the professionals. Nevertheless, I went, on the 4th of November.

The oncology department at The Royal Free Hospital is probably much like any other. When I entered and was directed to the waiting room, I found a large lounge with big doors that opened intermittently for patients to come and go, either in their chairs or with drips. I saw frail, pale, hairless patients carrying bowls into which they would occasionally vomit. I sat with my husband on the plastic chairs, watching and remembering my previous battles and how I'd overcome so much. Fear gripped me, and I became terrified that this was my future.

The previous week, I had endured my second visit to the breast clinic. Upon remembering this, I decided, right there in the waiting room, that I couldn't go through with it. I told Mohammad that I was discharging myself, but he said, since we were already there, we might as well hear what they had to say. So, we did.

Shortly thereafter, I was greeted by a tall doctor who said, "Well, we know what's wrong with you." I was momentarily shocked but proceeded with the ultrasound he insisted on. "Ah," my doctor said, "It's 5.5, not 6 centimetres." Clearly, he thought there had been a mistake in the original measurement. But I instantly knew that it had shrunk by 0.5 centimetres, and that was my sign that I was doing the right thing.

We sat back down, and the doctor said, "Right, you know what we're doing, don't you? I'm booking the double mastectomy as we speak." It all felt surreal. That was part of my body he was talking about cutting away, and it didn't feel like I had any choice. He told me I'd need both of my underarms cleared, not just one, just in case, and he mentioned that I'd always have problems using my arms afterward.

Again, I felt the waves of negativity barrelling towards me; I don't know how I was keeping my head above water. Mohammad silently sat next to me, the weight of it all pressing heavily on us both. I couldn't raise my gaze from the floor, nor blink my tears away quickly enough. The doctor continued regardless, going through my treatment plan, which included many rounds of harsh chemotherapy, followed by potential radiotherapy. The whole conversation felt as transactional as a chef reciting the ingredients of a recipe to an apprentice.

Somehow, I found inner strength and asked the doctor if he had finished. He told me he almost had, that he was just making a referral. I said, "No. I'm going!" I told him I was discharging myself, and he appeared shocked, telling me I couldn't. I argued, "I can, this is my body, and I can do what I please." The doctor, now panicking, asked me to speak with his senior, and reluctantly, I agreed.

Shortly after, a woman entered the room with the first doctor and introduced herself as the head of oncology. She said, "I'm sorry to hear about all your bad news." This was the first bit of sympathy I had received, but she quickly added, "I can see both you and your husband are upset, but we need to go through this treatment, the right treatment; we do this every day, and people come out fine afterwards." This struck me as absurd. I'd been told time and again that I would not come out of this fine, and I wanted to know how she was so sure this was the right treatment because I didn't agree.

I stood up, looking her straight in the eye, my own eyes red and sore, and I stood my ground. I restated that I was discharging myself, to which she replied, "Do you know what you're doing?" I answered honestly, "No, but I do know that I don't want to do what you're asking me to do." I left the room and then the hospital.

As far as I was concerned, I was on my own.

The Fight: On My Terms

I returned home after the oncology appointment, determined to prove them wrong. I had my discharge papers, my support network, and my instincts, so I knew they wouldn't need to bother me again. The breast clinic, however, was another matter. I was virtually bombarded with communications from them requesting reviews, but I just carried on fighting on my terms, driven by this inner voice.

Eventually, I decided to go back for another appointment at the breast clinic, around August, the year after my diagnosis. By that time, I had completely changed my lifestyle, having spent six months working intensely on myself. I'd been juicing and found fresh ginger and turmeric particularly useful, without fully understanding why. I learned why later, but at the time, I was content to trust my instincts to do the right thing, and I was increasingly feeling better as I expanded my knowledge and tried new things. Of course, I had the occasional negative thought, but I learned quickly to avoid that kind of thinking and keep focused.

I self-examined once a week, and as the weeks went by, I could feel my tumour getting smaller. At one point, spurred on by my own progress, I made a jar containing fresh ginger, garlic, turmeric, and olive oil. I'd created a kind of elixir that I felt I needed to take each day (just a spoonful) after my meals. It wasn't pleasant, but I believed it could help me, and that belief was important.

After juicing for around six months, the day of my breast clinic appointment—the six-month review—arrived on the 25th of August. I spent a lot of time that day reflecting on what had brought me to that point, and I began to wonder if the HRT and the lack of monitoring while taking it were the cause of the cancer. I was 43 when I started HRT on the advice of medics following my hysterectomy, and everything had seemed fine. But the lack of reviews over all those years gave me pause for thought. I also thought about self-neglect and wondered if the stress of my desire to heal and help others, putting my own needs last, had contributed to my ill health. Looking back, I realised I hadn't really ever shown myself much love or taken enough time for my own healing.

This time, at the breast clinic, my doctor wasn't able to see me, but I went in anyway and had my scan straight away. Instantly, I saw the young radiographer's eyes light up. She turned to me with surprise and asked, "What have you been doing?" I had done so much, I didn't know where to start, but I told her briefly about the juicing. She told me, "Well, whatever you've done is amazing. It's reduced the size by 1.5 centimetres, and the inflammation around it has completely settled."

I went on to see a female consultant afterwards, and that hope within me stirred once again, hoping she would agree that all was going to be fine. The reality, of course, was different. The consultant also asked me what I'd been doing and acknowledged that the reduction in size was good, but she still wanted to start me on 2.5mg of Letrozole, which I would have to take daily for the rest of my life as a preventative measure. I asked her why, if the danger seemed to be reducing, and her answer hit me like a blow to the chest. She told me, "Don't forget, your mum died of cancer." Straight away, that altered my thinking—how could it not? And sadly, I began to doubt myself. I agreed to take the tablets.

Back at home, that visit stayed with me for about a week. Then, despite having researched the side effects of the medication they wanted me to take (and finding them worrying), I felt so tired and so beaten down by the enormous pressure and relentless negativity that surrounded me that I acquiesced. I lay down and did as I was told.

Unfortunately, that brief period of a few months when I gave in and took the medication, which I knew deep down might harm me, caused a rise in blood pressure, blood sugars, and cholesterol, and ruined my joints—all known side effects I had read about. I couldn't believe it; I had made myself sicker! Obviously, I stopped taking the medicine and returned to caring for my body with methods that felt right to me, such as juicing and incorporating medicinal foods into my meals—methods I truly believed in.

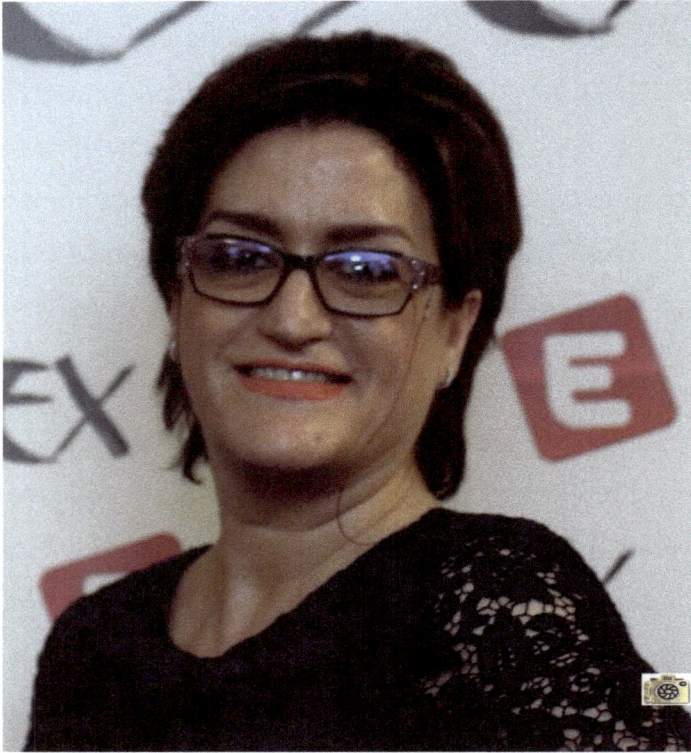

Celebrating hard-earned success in the media.
A photo shoot at Sussex radio, in London, in 2019.

The medical routes and interventions had not been right for my body, and I don't regret turning my back on them at all. But only recently have I come to understand that I will be okay, as I have developed a deeper understanding of my patterns of thinking and the power they hold.

Hossein's good friend, Matt Hudson, who also knows me very well, explained to me the concept of *Split-second Unlearning*, and I quickly realised what Hossein had done for me during that very early phone call we'd shared. First, from the medical professionals, I'd learned that I was going to die, but then I had unlearned this when Hossein made me see that there could be another way. If he hadn't done this, if no one else had managed to break through to me or had accepted my fate as it was delivered, I would very likely not have survived my cancer. *Split-second Unlearning* changed my entire pathway and set me on the road to recovery before I'd even tasted a salad leaf.

Matt writes…

'To understand Split-second Unlearning, we must first look at split-second learning or what behavioural psychologist Edwin Ray Guthrie termed 'contiguity learning'. Guthrie's theory states that all learning is based on a stimulus-response association, which lends itself to one-trial learning. His work remained unproven within the classroom learning environment, where for example we may have to practice equations in the math class or rehearse a poem over and over before committing it to memory. However, from the position of behavioural psychology 'contiguity learning' makes perfect sense and may well be the basis for many phobias, allergies, mental and physiological conditions.

**To the cancer that changed my life for the better...
I'm Still Here!**

Simple examples of contiguity learning can be the first time you burn your finger on a flame or hot surface, the experience is painful, and your mind learns in a split-second to avoid fire in the future. You don't need any more repetition to grasp the lesson from your first experience.

Emotional memory images are held inside the mind's eye, acting like psychological barriers to learning. Whenever they are activated the bodies fight, flight, freeze response system is activated. The challenge facing many people with psychophysiological dis-ease or illness is that the mind creates amnesia of the original event, so they are unaware of the emotional memory image that is causing their lack of energy, pain or hormonal imbalance.

Stress has been nominated as a key cause/component of many mental and physical health conditions, yet it is critical to realise that stress is a symptom, not a cause. What if emotional memory images are triggering your stress response and eroding your immune system?'

Matt's theory has stayed with me and has not only informed my professional practice but also serves as a reminder of my own power and influence over the course of my life.

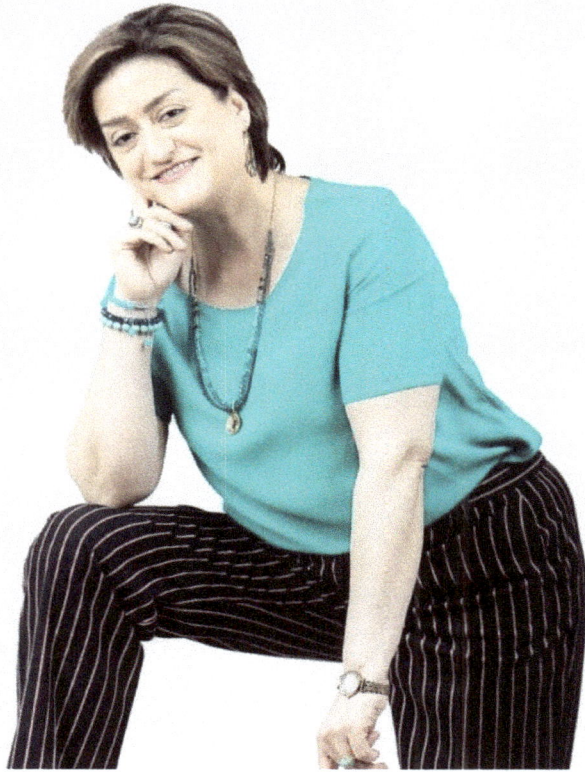

No matter what, I approach life with a smile on my face!

To The Cancer
That Changed My Life For The Better…

Dear cancer,

Thankfully, I am nearly seven years free of you now. But cancer, you have sat me down and taught me lessons that will stay with me for a lifetime.

I have learned…

The importance of looking after myself—a basic statement that is far easier to say than to put into action. Before you interrupted things, cancer, I spent so much time trying to heal and help others, as I believe I was born to do. But for most of my life, I was always in competition with myself to do better and to get better. I neglected myself, physically and emotionally. I did not value time to be with myself, and I did not stop to appreciate what I already had and what the world around me had to offer.

Now, I am my priority. I am kind to myself in the same way I am kind to my patients, and I nurture my connection with nature, which has made my life infinitely richer.

Lesson Number Two

Before you came along, cancer, I was scared of death; I really feared loss and I knew its pain. Now, I see things differently. I know that we are energy, and that energy never truly dies—it simply changes over time. So, when I lose loved ones, each one is still a loss, but instead of being devastated, I choose to see the beauty in the life that was lived, to cherish the memories I have of them, and to be grateful for their impact on my own being. And before I reach my own death, I will live a rich and full life.

Lesson Number Three

I am strong and powerful. When I needed to be, I was the BIG 'F' to your small 'c'. I faced you and I beat you back on my terms! Ultimately, I see now that I am responsible for all of the choices I have made in my lifetime, both the good and the bad, and that makes me an incredible force to be reckoned with. I carry this belief forward, and when faced with any illness or challenge, I tower over them with my strength and convictions; they are small and weak, and I am victorious! I know that a strong mind and self-belief are the first things you need when battling against the odds, because our beliefs shape our actions, and our actions are powerful.

Lesson Number Four

I deserve better. I deserve calmness, contentment, inner peace, and happiness in their purest forms. This belief was missing before you came along. To see me back then, smiling and dancing to the music in the background, you'd have thought I was the happiest girl in the world, but I needed so much input to feel that way. Now, I don't need to do anything at all. I am so full of unconditional love—for myself, for nature, for people—and I am so at peace, anywhere, at any time, that I attract love into my life every day, and I share it.

Lesson Number Five

You taught me that you do not determine my fate. I do. But I have learned that everyone, not just those struck by cancer, needs to hear that there is always hope and that they are not powerless. Now, I dedicate my life to helping people realise this, and part of doing that is in writing this book.

Cancer, about two years ago, in the latter half of 2022, when I came to accept that my beliefs and attitude shaped my path to recovery, I became even more of a force to be reckoned with. I believed I could treat myself, I believed I could beat you, and I believed, wholeheartedly, in the steps I took to do it. And didn't I show you?!

It is sobering to think that if I'd left the hospital in agreement with the team about my treatment plan, accepting my five-year potential survival rate, I could have laid down and lost my life to you, cancer. The experience still sends shivers down my spine. But now, I'm proud to say I've learned from all of the challenges I've faced in my life, including you. I've reframed them and see them all as opportunities for growth.

And I'm happier than I've ever been!

Yours Sincerely,

Fatemeh

**To the cancer that changed my life for the better…
I'm Still Here!**

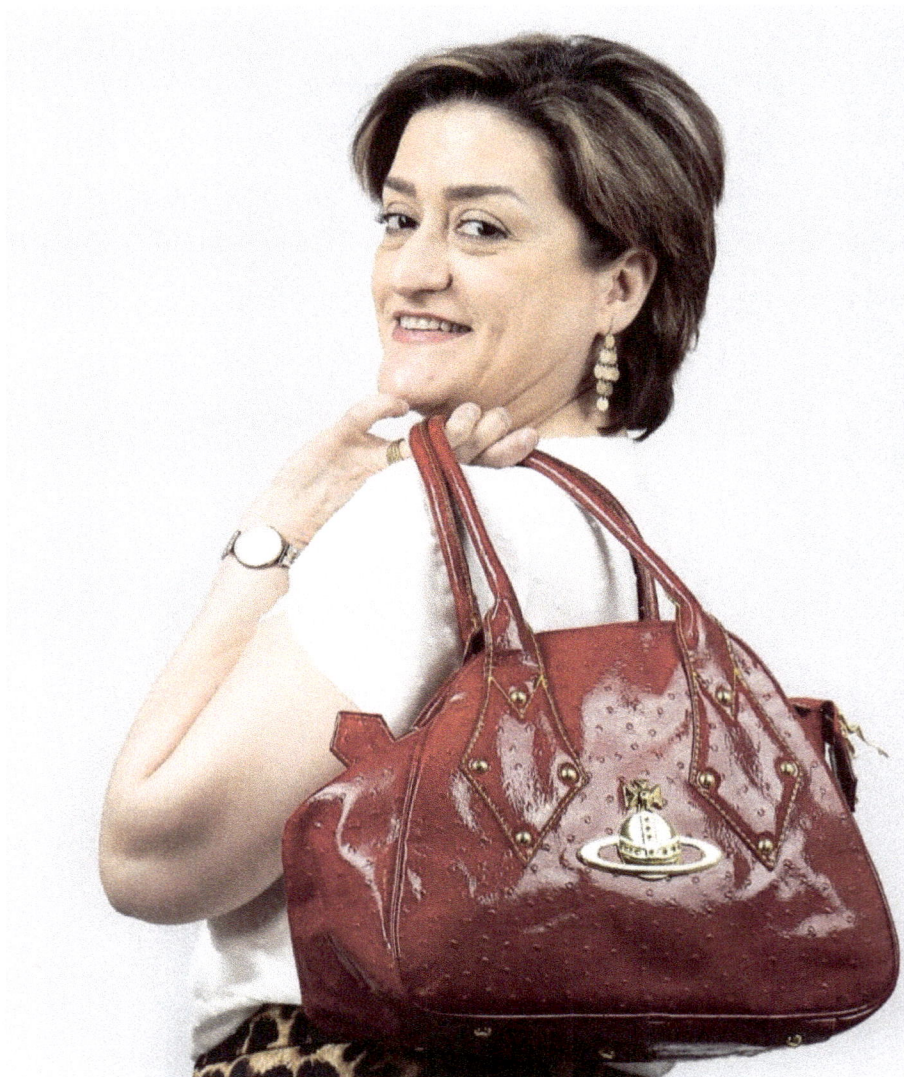

I have learnt my lessons,
I packed my knowledge and I am ready to share it with the world!

Acknowledgements

Matt Hudson, from Northeast England, is a social scientist and behavioural change consultant with 30 years of experience in private practice, specialising in the causes of psychophysiological disease. He ran a training company for 25 years, teaching hypnotherapy, Neuro-linguistic Programming (NLP), and his own theory, academically known as Split-Second Unlearning (SSU). Matt has published two peer-reviewed academic papers and has written extensively on the effects that fear can have on the human mind and body. His latest book, *Family Rules Okay*, explores systemic family systems. Since 2019, Matt has worked tirelessly to incorporate his method into a mental health app, MindReset. This evidence-based app uses eye-tracking technology to locate fear, clear it, and boost energy.

Salad Photo by Nadine Primeau
https://unsplash.com/s/photos/salad?utm_source=unsplash&utm_mediu m=referral&utm_content=creditCopyText

To the cancer that changed my life for the better…
I'm Still Here!

From the bottom of my heart, thank you to my wonderful family and friends – those who have been there for me, who have done more than they'll ever know. I am truly grateful.

And to my one true love, my incredible Mohammad - we did it…

I'm Still Here!

But, wait…

Dr Fatemeh isn't finished yet…

You can find out more about Dr. Fatemeh, get physiotherapy inspiration, interactive courses, tips, and even DVDs at www.drfatemeh.co.uk

www.ingramcontent.com/pod-product-compliance
Lightning Source LLC
Chambersburg PA
CBHW051248020426
42333CB00025B/3112